Caring for the
Psychogeriatric Client

Priscilla Ebersole, Ph.D., R.N. is Professor of Nursing at San Francisco State University. Her teaching assignments focus on mental health, geropsychiatric, and holistic nursing. Dr. Ebersole recently directed a 13-state project to recruit, educate, support, and integrate gerontological nurse practitioners in nursing homes. The project was funded by the W.K. Kellogg Foundation and administered by the Mountain States Health Corporation in Boise, Idaho. In the Fall of 1988 she occupied the Florence Cellar Endowed Chair in Gerontological Nursing at Case Western Reserve University. Dr. Ebersole has published extensively. She has twice received the AJN Book of the Year Award. Throughout 15 years of gerontologic interest and care, she has sustained a deep personal interest in the therapeutic aspects of reminiscing.

Caring for the Psychogeriatric Client

Priscilla Ebersole, Ph.D., R.N.

SPRINGER PUBLISHING COMPANY
New York

Springer Publishing Company, Inc.
536 Broadway
New York, NY 10012

89 90 91 92 93/5 4 3 2 1

Library of Congress Cataloging-in-Publication Data

Ebersole, Priscilla.
    Caring for the psychogeriatric client / Priscilla Ebersole.
        p.   cm.
    Bibliography: p.
    Includes index.
    ISBN 0-8261-6420-X
    1. Geriatric psychiatry.   2. Aged—Mental health services.
I. Title.
    [DNLM:D   1. Health Services for the Aged—organization &
administration.   2. Mental Disorders—in old age.   3. Mental
Disorders—therapy.   WT 150 E16c]
    RC451.4.A5E24   1989
    618.97'689—dc20
    DNLM/DLC
    for Library of Congress   89-11516
                                                                              CIP

Printed in the United States of America

Contents

v

Common Patient Management Problems • Communicating with the Stroke (CVA) Patient • Perseverative Communication • Sexual Acting Out • Wandering • Passivity • Disturbed Sleep Patterns • Falls • Incontinence • Eating Disorders

Preface

This text is designed for nurses, social workers, counselors, paraprofessionals, and community agency personnel who deal directly with the mental health needs and emotional disorders of the aged. The main emphasis is on management strategies shown effective with aged persons demonstrating a variety of emotional and behavioral problems. It is based upon current research and approaches reported as successful. The exigencies of providing care are approached in a realistic manner, knowing that ideal situations exist very rarely.

The objectives of the book are to:

Provide current knowledge related to the recognition and management of the mental and emotional problems of the aged.

Improve the capacity of professionals to deliver appropriate and humanistic care to the mentally and emotionally disturbed elder.

Foster motivation toward a focus on the quality of life for clients in their later years and their caregivers.

Encourage those who work with the disturbed aged to question the present state of the art and generate research aimed at more adequate management of their care.

When useful, diagnostic terms of the Diagnostic Statistical Manual (DSM III R), Psychiatric Nursing Diagnoses (PND), and North American Nursing Diagnostic Association (NANDA) have been incorporated into the book. Practical suggestions and ideas are presented for the life enrichment of the elders who are our predecessors on the journey into aging. Questions are raised to stimulate further research regarding the management of the mental health of the aged.

The book includes most of the common issues that must be understood in order to provide humanistic and holistic care, grounded in the belief that quality of life for caregivers and the aged is our highest goal in gerontic care. The book is slanted toward nursing and long-term care as these professionals deal most intimately and on a continuing basis with the emotional disturbances of elders. One chapter is also devoted to geropsychiatric disorders that account for most short-term hospitalizations and another chapter to the dynamics and needs of family caregivers. The principles and suggestions throughout the book can be extrapolated to acute care and community settings and may form the basis for more holistic care of the emotionally disturbed elder in whatever settings they are found.

At present, biomedical research, which consumes the lion's share of the research dollar in aging, has yet to address the daily management and concerns of the aged and those who care for them. Much of the research in aging has addressed the etiology and description of cognitive decrements and the dementias that afflict some aged. This is necessary for the future hope of cure but those presently afflicted and the ones who care for them must find their way with few clear directives. It is also important not to give the preponderance of dementia research more credence than is accurate in terms of the actual aging experience. Aging is a stage of development about which we have yet much to learn. If we limit our perspective to that of decrements, we will address aging only as a medical problem. While this book is designed to assist caregivers to deal with emotional problems that are often a concomitant of the aging experience, it is important not to forget that the aged are our greatest resource. In the problems of living, they are the masters and we the students. We must be willing to learn from them. However, because of the love of youth that is so inherent in our society, we often neglect the validity of aging. As a result, some issues addressed in this book are related to the broader perspective of ageism as a social phenomenon.

In this book, I have tried to induce wonder and a sense of awe toward those of our predecessors who have survived the vicissitudes of the past seven to eight decades. When we see those who embody our past and portend our future, we must continually examine our approaches to their care lest we study their adaptation and think, in our innocence, that we understand the history and demands that they have experienced.

In other words, our legitimate concern with the daily experience of the aged, of their coping and survival, form the background and possibility for a richer and fuller life experience for each of us. Let us not look on the disturbances of old age with disdain. We are all traveling the continuum of life. Working with the elderly provides an opportunity to be cognizant of life in all its adaptations and diversity, to know its gifts, and to accept the full spectrum of human attributes.

1

An Introduction to Psychogeriatric Care

The aged in our society who are emotionally disturbed or mentally ill have been largely neglected. Perhaps the most prevalent of all ageist attitudes are toward these emotionally or mentally impaired elders. They are stigmatized and underserved. Few mental health professionals are educationally prepared to specialize in the care of the aged though many are doing so out of necessity. Some openly declare their preference for younger clients. Too often, traditional psychiatrists feel there is little purpose in extensive psychotherapy for an individual who has only a few years left to live. The aged themselves rarely seek treatment for mental or emotional disorders. As a society, we generally assume that the aged are less inclined to seek attention for what they consider problems of living that must simply be endured. Those who have cognitive disturbances may not have the motivation or awareness of the need for care until they are totally disabled. At this point, help is usually sought by the family. However, for those with limited resources, the expense of outpatient psychotherapy may be prohibitive and limitations in Medicare and Medicaid restrictive. For the vast majority of mentally and emotionally disturbed elders, the result has been inadequate care and inappropriate institutionalization usually in nursing homes where resources tend to be limited and mental health professionals least available.

CARE OF THE MENTALLY ILL AGED IN NURSING HOMES

Through Title IXX (Medicaid) and other legislation, federal policy has subverted long-term care for the mentally disturbed elderly. In 1950, Congress enacted legislation which defined settings primarily engaged in providing care of persons with mental disorders as Institutions for Mental Disease (IMDs). In addition, it has long been assumed that individual states were responsible for such care.

When, in the mid-1960s, federal policy mandated what seemed a more humane (and economic) policy of deinstitutionalization, legislation was enacted to exclude Medicaid reimbursement to facilities providing mental health services for more than half the residents. The rationale behind this focused on mental health services as a state responsibility. However, it soon became apparent that states were not prepared to care for the mentally ill in community settings. As a result, most of the aged mentally ill were simply moved from large to small asylums (nursing homes). Studies in Illinois, Utah, Massachusetts, and Texas show that 65% of intermediate care (ICF) residents are former mental patients and that Board and Care Homes and ICFs constitute the two long-term care settings in which most former mental patients reside. Many argue that the state institutions provided much more adequately for human needs and psychiatric care. Yet nursing homes are now the largest single setting for the care of the mentally ill elderly. More than three-quarter million elderly mentally ill reside in nursing homes, five times the number of mentally ill in state institutions (Harper, 1986). It is estimated that 60% of all nursing home residents suffer from a chronic mental condition. Accurate data cannot be obtained as primary diagnoses of nursing home residents are slanted toward reimbursement requirements and the general absence of psychological assessment in these settings.

Emotional, behavioral, and mental disorders frequently observed in nursing homes include depression, confusion, disorientation, wandering, restlessness, agitation, lethargy, irritability, stress, low self-esteem, guilt, delusions, paranoia, and inappropriate dependence on staff. In most cases, the care provided to resolve these problems is given by aides and orderlies who have neither the knowledge nor the skill to deal with them effectively. In addition, state and federal regulations do not *require* any care for mental problems specifically. Often, then, unless elderly residents who suffer from these problems disturb staff or other residents, the emotional issues remain unattended.

Only 20% of nursing home residents have a primary diagnosis of mental disorder (Harper, 1986). The remaining 80% may have undiagnosed disorders, secondary mental illness, or are "at risk" due to the effects of nursing home placement, physical impairments, the medical model of the milieu, and the restrictive life style.

Kramer et al. (in German & Kramer, 1986) devised a diagnostic interview schedule (DIS) based on the *Diagnostic and Statistical Manual (DSM) III* diagnoses to be used in greater Baltimore area nursing homes to determine psychiatric disorders among residents. All but one nursing home in the catchment area participated in the project. Distribution of diagnoses generated in the study can be seen in Table 1.1. Most interesting is the high incidence of phobics in the first year of admission to a nursing home. German and Kramer also found that almost 15% of residents diagnosed at admission to have mental impairment were normal when tested during the study. While there is a dearth of similar studies that could provide more nationally applicable data, this study provides food for thought.

TABLE 1.1   Current DIS Diagnosis by Length of Stay in Nursing Home

	Length of stay	
Current diagnosis	Less than 1 year	1 year or more
	(174–181)*	(104–144)*
Schizophrenia	0.6	0.7
Affective disorders	6.8	2.1
Phobias	11.6	2.1
Substance abuse or dependence	0.6	0.0
Antisocial personality	0.7	0.0
Other DIS disorders	3.3	0.7
Any DIS diagnosis	41.1	25.3
Cognitive impairment[+]	24.0	21.5

*These numbers represent the range of individuals for any single diagnosis. Certain diagnoses could not be made because of lack of information. Individuals could have more than one diagnosis however.

[+]Cognitive impairment here is based on the Mini-Mental State test administered to patients. It does not include chart diagnoses.

Source: German, P., & Kramer, M. (1986). Nursing home study of the Eastern Baltimore epidemiological catchment area study. In M. Harper & B. Lebowitz (Eds.), Mental Illness in Nursing Homes: Agenda for Research. U.S. Dept of Health & Human Services, Public Health Service Alcohol, Drug Abuse & Mental Health Administration.

Liptzin (1986) discusses four distinct categories of mental disorders found among nursing home residents: the chronic mentally ill, the chronic mentally disabled, chronic mental patients, and those with recent onset of psychiatric disturbance. The chronic mentally ill may have a classic diagnosis but yet manage functionally quite well. On the other hand, the chronic mentally disabled have severe impairment in functional ability while chronic mental patients are those who have been institutionalized for prolonged periods. Those patients with recent onset of problems merit intensive effort as their psychiatric problems are likely to be reversible. Most frequent of these disorders can be seen in Table 1.2.

The vast majority (80%) of nursing homes are operated for profit (National Center for Health Statistics, 1983). The development of large corporate interests in nursing homes was facilitated by the tax, real estate, and administrative structures imposed related to management and reimbursement (German & Kramer, 1986). Small family-owned operations have largely been phased out or bought up. Major deficiencies in nursing homes most often cited include untrained and inadequate staff, few activities, profiteering, lack of respect for human dignity, overreliance on drugs, unsanitary conditions, unauthorized use of restraints, negligence leading to injury or death, theft, and untrained administrators. While enormous improvements have been made in many facilities, there is still much to do to create satisfying and therapeutic environments in nursing homes. The need for nursing homes is predicted to increase despite the development of day care, home health, and other care options. As health professionals, we have a serious responsibility to our elders, and our elder selves, to make these facilities *homes* in which the holistic needs of residents are a high priority.

STAFFING FOR PSYCHOGERIATRIC CARE

Staffing for psychogeriatric care varies greatly depending on the setting in which the client receives care. Within geropsychiatric hospital units, nurses and mental health paraprofessionals provide most of the direct care under the guidance and direction of a psychiatrist. In some fortunate situations, there are geropsychiatric nurse specialists and geropsychiatric physicians available. Psychiatric social workers are integral to the professional team and provide case management, resource information, and family support. Neurologists, internists, geriatricians, and clinical psychologists are also essential to the adequate diagnosis and management of patient care. Fortunately, as of April

TABLE 1.2 Four Most Frequent DIS/DSM-III Psychiatric Disorders,* by Rank, Sex, and Age, Based on 6-Month Prevalence Rates

	Age group				
Rank	18–24	25–44	45–64	65+	Total
Male					
1	Alcohol abuse/ dependence	Alcohol abuse/ dependence	Alcohol abuse/ dependence	Severe cognitive impairment	Alcohol abuse/ dependence
2	Drug abuse/ dependence	Phobia	Phobia	Phobia	Phobia
3	Phobia	Drug abuse/ dependence	Dysthymia	Alcohol abuse/ dependence	Drug abuse/ dependence
4	Antisocial personality	Antisocial personality	Major depressive episode without grief	Dysthymia	Dysthymia
Female					
1	Phobia	Phobia	Phobia	Phobia	Phobia
2	Drug abuse/ dependence	Major depressive episode without grief	Dysthymia	Severe cognitive impairment	Major depressive episode without grief
3	Major depressive episode without grief	Dysthymia	Major depressive episode without grief	Dysthymia	Dysthymia
4	Alcohol abuse/ dependence	Obsessive compulsive disorder	Obsessive compulsive disorder	Major depressive episode without grief	Obsessive compulsive disorder

*Dysthymia included. The basis for ranking was the mean 6-month prevalence rates for New Haven, Baltimore, and St. Louis combined. DIS indicates Diagnostic Interview Schedule.

Taube, R., & Barrett, J. (1986). Mental Health in the United States, 1985. National Institutes of Mental Health, United States Dept of Health & Human Services. Washington, D.C. U.S. Government Printing Office.

1988 the American Medical Association (AMA) began certifying geriatricians so that physicians qualified to care for the aged can now be identified. There are also increasing numbers of geropsychiatric clinical nurse specialists who are clearly well qualified for all but the medical management of psychogeriatric clients. Because they currently form the most available of fully qualified geropsychiatric professionals, their role and capacities will be discussed in some depth.

Within the community, clients are most often managed by nurses in consultation with an agency or hospital-based team of professionals similar to those described above. Some geriatric assessment teams that provide services in the home include psychologists, social workers, geriatric nurse practitioners, physicians, and rehabilitation specialists of various types. However, these full-team services to the home are infrequent. Geriatric nurse practitioners are, however, becoming more visible in community care in clinics and in home care. Geriatric nurse practitioners are able to provide comprehensive care that will be discussed later in the chapter.

In long-term care, the situation is much different. There is a dearth of professionals and in some settings registered nurses (RNs) are only available on the day shift. Most care is provided by licensed vocational nurses, aides, and orderlies. Particular services of social workers, psychiatric nurses, psychologists, rehabilitation specialists, and psychiatrists are often on a consultant basis only and far too infrequently used. Because of the great need in the majority of these settings, special attention has been given throughout this text to caring for the emotionally disturbed elder in a long-term care setting. Undoubtedly, the psychogeriatric clinical nurse specialist and the geriatric nurse practitioner have significant potential for improving the situation in these settings.

Geropsychiatric Clinical Nurse Specialists

The geropsychiatric clinical nurse specialist (GCNS) is a professional prepared to work within any setting serving the emotional needs of elders and can offer administrative, clinical, educational, and research expertise. Behavior problems, whether secondary to the stress of institutionalization or significant pathology, are the responsibility of nursing management. The knowledge base of the GCNS reflects a thorough understanding of normal and abnormal changes of aging, judicious use of psychotropic medications, and developmental issues of late life. Although this role within nursing is relatively new, it is an important step in meeting the critical need for mental health services in the nursing home setting (Eliasberg, 1987).

Geriatric patients with behavioral problems in acute- and long-term care facilities require vast amounts of staff time. Early detection and treatment of problems such as dementia, depression, agitation, paranoia, delusions, and hallucinations will benefit patient, staff, and family. The psychogeriatric clinical nurse specialist, who receives supervision from a consulting psychiatrist, can facilitate early detection and diagnosis. Other functions of this nurse are to provide indirect consultation to staff, suggest management strategies, evaluate and follow up on the effectiveness of interventions, provide educational offerings for all disciplines, suggest applications of current research as it applies to the setting, and conduct nursing research. Particular issues that may require formal and informal staff conferences include pain control, adjustment to illness, hospitalization, nursing home placement, and preparation for death.

To meet current needs, which can be termed *desperate* in some settings, the role of the geropsychiatric nursing specialist must be enhanced. Remember, these nurses may provide much needed consultation, staff support, and patient counseling. While there are a limited number of these nurses presently educated, their numbers exceed those of geropsychiatrists. In addition, they are much more likely to be interested in working in long-term care. Unfortunately, in this era of economic constraint, the expanding need for geriatric psychiatric services is most vulnerable to continuing neglect. To counter such prospects, directors of nursing service must take the initiative in insisting that such services are or become available. In the long term, the cost of these additional services would be well offset by reduced stress on caregivers and greater psychological and functional satisfaction among patients.

In a veterans hospital, for example, a geropsychiatric clinical specialist fills several roles (O'Conner, 1987). He or she formulates various group strategies to meet specific resident needs, directs groups, and educates staff in these group techniques. Other components of the role include managing the difficult patient, negotiating control issues of staff and patient autonomy, directing regular problem-solving sessions with staff, providing in-service educational sessions routinely, and providing direct care by acting as intermediary in confrontive issues with staff and residents.

Creative staffing patterns may be needed to meet the physical and psychological needs of psychogeriatric patients. However, the need to provide physical care may leave little time to intervene with the patient's psychological needs. Some of these physical care and functional tasks can be delegated to nursing assistants hired for specific blocks of time in which functional needs are highest, such as early morning, mealtimes, and bedtime.

Geriatric Nurse Practitioners

The geriatric nurse practitioner (GNP) is prepared, usually through Master's degree preparation, to provide comprehensive and sophisticated management of health problems encountered by aged clients. Geriatric nurse practitioners work in concert with physicians but are often the primary managers in long-term care. The legal constraints of their function vary from state to state. In some states they are given prescriptive privileges and may be directly reimbursed for services. Overall, in long-term care settings, they have had a marked impact on the quality of physical and psychosocial care.

The most recent extensive study of the cost and qualitative effectiveness of geriatric nurse practitioners was carried out by Kane et al. (1988). Though the results were not as strong as anticipated, the study showed that in areas of patient and family satisfaction, reduced reliance on transfer to acute care, and illness resolution the presence of GNPs resulted in more positive outcomes. The pervasive effects of GNP staffing indicate an overall general shift toward a more satisfactory milieu in which they are integral members of staff. In addition, morale of other staff and patients is affected by the immediately available services of a GNP when problems occur. Because they have a knowledgeable resource person at their disposal, staff feel less helpless. Patients are grateful that their health needs can be assessed immediately and appropriate action taken. Many of the emotional reactions to delay in having needs attended to can also be averted, another significant gain. Some of the particular benefits of GNPs not addressed in the Kane et al. study (1988) include reduction in staff turnover, reduced numbers of citations for inadequate care, and census predictability at higher levels. While GNPs have a less extensive background in psychogeriatric care than psychogeriatric clinical specialists, their ability to astutely determine physical ramifications of observable problems makes them invaluable to the caregiving team.

Developing Staff Attitudes and Expertise

Staffing in geropsychiatric and long-term care units requires particular consideration. Staff persons often become pseudo-family and develop strong and meaningful relationships with patients. Nursing staff frequently state the reason for selecting long-term care is associated with the possibility and quality of relationships that exist in those settings (Ebersole, 1986). By accepting the validity and frequency of this underlying motivation, it seems reasonable to plan to enhance possibilities. Miller (1986) studied the development of relationships in

long-term care and found that despite heavy work loads, close relationships are formed between the majority of nursing assistants and
some of their patients. They also noted that both patient and nurse
showed greater life satisfaction and physical and mental health when
this occurred. Impediments to such relationships were usually embedded in previously held negative stereotypes and could be effectively combated with experiential exercises.

In 1984 a particularly effective way of promoting significant relationships between caregivers and patients was instituted in the Hillhaven nursing homes (Troyer, 1984). Each person working in the
nursing home, from administrator to janitor, is encouraged to
"Adopt-a-resident" to whom they give special attention and some
time each day. Craven (1988) reports that some of these commit-
ments develop into long, intimate, and very human relationships.

A particularly creative program to enhance the psychosocial abilities of Certified Nursing Assistants (CNAs) was instituted in a Maine
nursing home (Bayer, Bresloff, & Curley, 1986). Once every 10 days,
each CNA is given a special assignment in which he or she is not
allowed to give any physical care. Rather the CNA is to focus entirely
on psychosocial care and communication. Specific activities that
might engage the CNA include writing letters for the patient, participating with patients in recreational therapy, participating in small
group work with patients, and developing a patient's life history. In
the morning, the CNA meets with the Director of Nursing Service
(DNS), Social Service (SS), and Recreational Therapist (RT) to plan
the day's activities. At the end of the day, the CNA meets with a
supervisor to discuss strategies, reactions, and knowledge gained. The
CNA also reads assigned articles and keeps a personal journal of
feelings. As a result of this program, staff morale was affected in a
positive manner: each CNA looked forward to his or her "day" to
focus on the more humanistic needs of their patients. In addition, all
staff involved in the program displayed increased patient awareness,
self-confidence, and sensitivity to patient feelings. Though the article
did not comment on the enhancement of relationships, it would be
interesting to investigate this aspect in a replication of the program.

Meeting the Staff Needs of Psychogeriatric Patients

Meeting the staff needs of the psychogeriatric patient in the acute-care
setting can be extremely difficult. With the significant increase in the
population of elderly clients, there is an obvious need for special
assessment and intervention although trained personnel and adequate
facilities may not be available. To counteract this more common

situation, a psychogeriatric educational program might be offered and actively promoted by the staff development office in each acute-care hospital. Learning goals would be focused on early detection of psychiatric problems and preventive strategies for those at risk and for those with developing problems.

As a general rule, mental health training programs for nursing home staff are integral to the development of appropriate nursing care plans to meet the actual needs of patients. Only 11% of all nursing home employees are registered nurses. It is imperative, therefore, that education programs be provided for nursing assistants who actually provide the majority of hands-on care. Baldwin (1987) developed a modularized training program that included didactic components each week followed by application and consultation with geropsychiatric nursing clinical specialists. Didactic modules included:

Stress management of caregivers.
Attitudes and myths regarding aging.
Dealing with aggressive behaviors.
Understanding dementias.
Understanding mental illness.
Enhancing residents' self-esteem.
Therapeutic interventions with families and friends.

All levels of nursing staff attended and each experience was designed to address their individual learning needs.

Training Nursing Assistants

Case studies are a particularly effective learning strategy for the education of nursing assistants in the management of patients' emotional and behavioral difficulties. The frequent and prolonged contact they have with patients can be most influential in the success of therapeutic efforts. In addition, the success of care plans are entirely dependent on the involvement, commitment, and abilities of the nursing assistants who must activate them. Weber and McCall (1987) note that as there are few large blocks of time for training these individuals, short, directed discussions of practical case situations can be most productive. Case discussions should include relevant questions such as:

What actually happened in this case?
What were the precipitants, or what led up to it?
What were the staff feeling and thinking?

What were they trying to accomplish?
What did the nursing assistant do?
What was effective and what was not effective?
What alternative actions might have been employed?

Insights and new approaches to care must be actively sought for nursing assistants. The nursing home can, through thoughtful attention to the education of nursing assistants, create a "therapeutic community" in which everyday routines and relationships contribute to residents' well-being.

Conversely, those who are exposed to overwhelming patient needs for prolonged periods without adequate means of assisting the patient will become callous and indifferent to them. At best, care of the chronically impaired is stressful for aides and orderlies who are paid minimal wages and often receive little recognition for the difficult work they do. Haley (1987), for example, addressed this problem by studying the psychosocial variables that were thought to affect burnout of nonprofessional staff. Significant factors that prevented burnout were found in the level of social and work support perceived by the individual. Surprisingly, length of service in the facility did not seem to be a significant factor.

A nursing assistant needs a number of skills to work well with the elderly. One of the most important is the ability to recognize and encourage patients to use their strengths. Some suggestions for doing so are given by Weber and McCall (1987):

Offering presence and reliable human contact.
Ensuring dignity by being courteous, considerate, and paying attention to the resident.
Involving residents in all possible decisions.
Making suggestions for courses of action while respecting the individual's right to refuse.
Giving direct orders only when essential for protection of self or others.
Encouraging the expression of feelings and accepting them in a nonjudgmental manner.
Patiently and clearly providing reality orientation.

St. George and DiCicco-Bloom (1986) have suggested that particularly difficult problems faced by staff may be managed through structured improvisation. This method allows staff to rehearse various ways of dealing with problems before they present. Suggested events that may need to be dramatized as provided in the list below. Ideally, these various approaches to problems could be videotaped for self-critique and elaboration by other staff.

PROBLEM BEHAVIORS

Management Through Structured Improvisation
Dramatic events such as:
  Coping with alcoholic behavior
  Sexual acting out
  Loss of roommate
  Racial prejudice
  Dying patients
  Conflict management
  Confusion/disorientation
Encourage feedback from actor and trainee.
Goal: To expand understanding and coping skills of staff.
  To enhance feelings of capability and effectiveness
  in managing difficult situations.

St. George & DiCicco-Bloom, NO 1986

There is the hope, of course, that these approaches will increase awareness of optional alternatives to patient care for nursing assistants and will encourage feedback and discussion among staff. In the end, such activity has two goals: (1) to enhance feelings of effectiveness and (2) to reinforce positive outcomes.

Clergy

Clergy may be significant in the management of mental health problems of aging. Indeed, some emotional disturbances may arise from spiritual conflicts or confrontation with values and uncertainties in the face of impending death. A sample of 1,135 older adults in Illinois showed greater levels of subjective well-being as measured by the Philadelphia Geriatric Center Morale Scale when involved in religious activities of organizational or nonorganizational nature. This was particularly true of women (Koenig, 1987).

Unfortunately, in nonsectarian nursing homes the role of clergy has not been given sufficient attention. To individuals indicating interest, however, the services clergy can provide are important. Weekly and biweekly services as well as last rites and spiritual counseling can be made available. In Toronto, for example, chaplains are available and supported by the city budget in metropolitan-owned facilities (Hilliard, 1987). While it is unlikely that most cities will support the services of chaplains in nursing homes, there are other ways to gain access to their services. Contacting the local office of the Council of Churches, or comparable organizations, to stimulate interest in serving elders in nursing homes is one avenue of immediate use.

Many individuals seek reconciliation with God and other persons as death approaches. Pain and other disabilities may interfere with this reconciliation. Symptomatic control in a milieu that responds to psychological, social, and religious needs can facilitate this process of adjustment. This requires a multidisciplinary team that includes pastoral care of the dying as a high priority. Schuman (1987) reports on such an undertaking that developed in response to the expressed needs of patients and families. Again, this approach deserves serious consideration: an individual must feel involved and in control of his or her treatment and care as long as life persists. Pastoral care seems to facilitate this humanistic approach.

Depressed elders often express concerns that have religious overtones. When this is the case, the need for pastoral counseling should be seriously considered and every effort made to assist the elder toward spiritual peace.

Mental Health of Staff

Given the prevalence of aides and orderlies as direct care providers in long-term care, it is incumbent on professionals and management to attend to their basic needs, psychic resources, and emotional health. Given the economic and time constraints administrators face, however, it is easiest to ignore this most basic foundation of good care. Those who are able to see the benefit in meeting staff needs will be amply repaid by lowered staff turnover, increased morale and motivation, and residents who function maximally.

Ways staff can be served to their benefit and that of the facility include:

• Purchasing of hard and soft goods at wholesale prices afforded by the institution.
• Weekly raffles of items donated by community merchants.
• Awards prominently displayed for individuals who develop special programs or activities.
• Day care facilities for children of staff members.

- Educational opportunities with time and pay coverage by the facility.
- Frequent meetings for staff to air concerns, feelings, and plan care.
- Individual counseling available to distressed staff members.
- Decision-making opportunities regarding facility needs and mangement.
- Academic affiliations.

DEVELOPING PSYCHOGERIATRIC CARE MODELS

Farran (1987) addressed issues in managing a psychogeriatric inpatient unit to maintain a therapeutic milieu. Responding to the medical as well as the psychiatric needs of clients necessitates creative staffing patterns and adequate preadmission assessment. Patient mix must also be given careful planning as one determines the effect an individual may have on the unit milieu. Maintaining a therapeutic milieu depends upon a carefully selected patient mix for each unit, based upon the patient's levels of cognition, mobility, and agitation. Each facility must decide how to make these determinations and what mix will be placed on each unit. The important factor to remember is this: based on the unique characteristics of staff and facility, give serious consideration both to staff stress and patient needs. Staff burnout can be avoided by such planning. A balance of nursing care hours must be plotted in order to care for all persons on the unit adequately. An important aspect of the milieu is the development and maintenance of a group program that is flexible and responsive to the unique needs of individual patients.

An appropriate and successful example of good psychogeriatric inpatient planning is offered by King (1987). In Ottawa, a psychogeriatric clinic has become a vital addition to services provided for elders. The clinic offers multidisciplinary assessment and treatment. Home assessments; followup visits; psychosocial, nursing, medication, and occupational therapy consultation are included in the comprehensive care plans. Referrals are accepted from anyone in the community. The clinic also provides consultation to nursing homes and ongoing support groups for elders at risk. These include such foci as relaxation, memory strengthening, and peer counseling.

Roy, Obaid, and Rudick (1987) report similar services provided in Middletown, New York, through a mobile geriatric treatment team. The team has been able to avert in-patient psychiatric hospitalization for 77% of cases seen. Comparable efforts in communities throughout the nation should certainly be given thoughtful consideration. Providing such services within the home is not only cost effective but more attendant to the holistic perspective of an individual's needs. Older persons account for only 5% of visits made to mental health clinics and less than 2% of visits to private psychotherapists (Nesbit, 1987). Given the realization that most elders seek their internist when encountering an emotional problem, it is imperative to employ acceptable and comprehensive methods of meeting their needs. The mobile mental health clinics seem a step in the right direction. Additionally, the identification of high-risk individuals, such as those living alone, homebound, recently bereaved, suffering repeated falls or hospitalizations and mental deterioration, and providing preventive supports could best be accomplished by a mobile mental health unit. Knight et al. (1982) has reported one such model in Ventura, California. Here, the services of a psychologist, nurses, geriatric nurse practitioner, and a psychiatrist provide individuals with comprehensive physical and mental health assessments and problem management.

A multidisciplinary behavioral neuropsychiatric unit has also been developed at Jewish Memorial Hospital in Boston to evaluate and modify behavioral problems that interfere with the elderly person's ability to function in the community. The staff are trained to eliminate inappropriate behavior by systematically reinforcing positive, appropriate behavior. Behaviors are carefully observed and recorded twice daily and discussed at a weekly planning session for modification of approach and evaluation of progress. Families are encouraged to participate in all aspects of the care plan. Results have been positive and suggest the applicability of the multidisciplinary behavioral management approach to dealing with troublesome behaviors (Lightfoot & To, 1989).

The following is a list of important criteria of excellence in geropsychiatric care:

Staff are interested in patients.
Former mental patients are housed separately from others.
The facility is clean.
Residents are actively involved with community.
Patients do not "act out" aggressively.
There is an activity program.
Staff turnover is low and staff like their jobs.
Food is adequate and nutritious.
Staff cooperates with outside agencies.
Staff have training to deal with psychiatric problems.
There is a high ratio of staff to patients.

Residents are neat and clean.
Patient care plans are appropriate and current.
Patients have private rooms.
Efforts are made toward independent living.
Active efforts are made to decrease problem behaviors.
Therapeutic and rehabilitation programs are available.

MENTAL HEALTH CONSULTATION

Levitan and Kornfeld (1981) have studied and advocated routine psychiatric consultation when elderly clients are admitted to the acute hospital for physical ailments, surgery, and fractures. The consultation focused on detecting and treating depression and postoperative delirium, if such existed, and advising staff and families in order to correct misimpressions of a poor prognosis. Those patients served by the consultants were discharged in two-thirds of the time of a similar control group and twice as many were returned home rather than being discharged to a nursing home.

Below is a case study that illustrates the benefits of psychiatric consultation.[1]

Sarah was an 88-year-old lady hospitalized for hip replacement surgery. The student psychiatric nurse attending her was expected to make a psychosocial assessment of her needs. The student was surprised at her wit, clarity, and cheerfulness, and concluded the client was coping well. The student remained with her throughout preparations for surgery and accompanied her to observe the surgery. Upon returning to the unit on the following day, the student found Sarah in total disarray, the bed littered with her personal belongings as if she were trying to pack; she was trying vainly to dial the telephone. Sarah also thought the nurses were trying to poison her and seemed frightened. Ideally, the student would have warned Sarah prior to surgery that people often have strange ideas, fears, and unrealistic thoughts following surgery. Since she had been so impressed by Sarah, she had not given adequate anticipatory guidance. At this point, it was difficult to break through the barrier of fear, confusion, and unreality. The interventions were devised to restore a sense of security and to reduce fear and environmental demands. The student remained with Sarah most of the morning and frequently reminded her that her thoughts were muddled as a result of the trauma of surgery but that she would soon regain her psychologic equilibrium. It was extremely important to continue reassuring Sarah that she was doing well and experiencing a temporary reaction due to surgery. Most of us have a deeply buried fear that we may "lose our mind." Sarah was greatly relieved to know she had not descended into a never-ending dementia. Though her thoughts remained mildly disordered for two more days,

[1] Throughout this volume, all case studies are derived from the author's personal experience unless otherwise indicated.

she completely recovered her cognitive capacity, wit, and cheerfulness as would be expected. Her family also needed considerable time to discuss their fears when confronted with the marked change in Sarah's personality. This is only one of many such cases in which outcomes are greatly affected by timely guidance and appropriate support (Ebersole, 1988).

Quite often, there is a reluctance to engage a psychiatrist in a case unless the symptoms are unmanageable. Clinicians are not nearly so loath to consider a spinal tap or a complete gastrointestinal (GI) series as an initial workup even though they are potentially harmful to a frail elder. However, many mental health centers have consultation teams that are readily available. It is high time that clinicians begin to use them preventively rather than only in crises.

Nursing Home Consultation

Nursing home consultation is frequently necessary to deal appropriately with management of disturbed patients. Though it may not be readily available, it is most often sought for aberrant behavior and affective disorders. Loebel (1987) found that in five Seattle nursing homes 25% of patients were given psychiatric referrals. Reasons for referral included:

Behavioral difficulties	32%
Weight loss and insomnia	13%
Depression/suicidality	20%
Psychiatric history	11%
Hallucinations and delusions	9%

Outcomes of psychiatric evaluation and recommendations by a nursing home consultation team resulted in 40% discharge rate with treatment goals attained within a year.

Consultation between nursing home and mental health centers also is available. The mental health centers across the nation have been designed to provide an array of services of varying intensity and diversity to the whole population within a geographically defined catchment area. In the 20 years since their inception, they have met the charge quite well in spite of budget restrictions, shifting social problems, and changing political ideologies. However, there is still much to be done in serving the aged. There are few geropsychiatrists and none that can be identified in most directories. Additionally, reimbursement restrictions through Medicare, with strict limitations on type and length of services, are barriers to full attention to the mental health of the aged. As a result of this situation, obtaining consultive services may be the most feasible manner of addressing mental health problems of the aged hospitalized, those receiving home care, and those in long-term care.

ASSESSMENT OF THE AGED

The need to assess older adults as unique individuals with particular problems related to their age and health is a serious undertaking. Indeed, as Terri and Lewinsohn (1986, xiii) state, the aged are "whole, complex beings and not oversimplified caricatures of a particular age or problem." A thoughtful assessment must begin with the examiner's awareness of his or her own attitudes and biases toward aging that may influence conclusions. In this regard, four critical considerations are fundamental to thorough assessment:

Each older adult must be viewed as a unique and complex being.
Adequate planning must be based in an interdisciplinary model and recognition of the need for specialized services.
Assessment data should be derived from multiple perspectives and sources.
Intrapersonal, interpersonal, and environmental factors in the setting that influence assessment and treatment planning must be carefully considered.

To ensure appropriate interventions, meticulous assessment is the first step. Even though each individual is unique, there are certain factors that are commonly considered in the assessment of the aged. See the boxed material.

SPECIAL CONSIDERATIONS IN ASSESSMENT OF THE AGED

Even subtle changes in biologic and psychosocial systems are often reflected in altered function, particularly of cognition.
Data concerning the aged can be easily skewed if not considered from a background of knowledge concerning his or her living situation, primary and secondary network, and support systems. This includes knowledge about the neighborhood in which the aged client lives and availability of sustaining services. Assessments of individuals in

hospitals and other institutions are at best limited. As a result, home assessments have been practiced by many geriatric assessment teams and often provide critical data that would otherwise be unavailable.

Nurses who spend more time with clients become cognizant of biorhythmic shifts that significantly alter assessment data depending upon time of day.

Significant others must be considered in any complete assessment. They are able to share valuable information.

Remember that the presenting problem may be of little significance to the elder. Find out what he or she thinks is most important.

Cohort factors (i.e., the historic period in which one is born and how that influences development) may also skew perception if not taken into account.

Fatigue and anxiety will erode performance. Sensitive or sophisticated assessments must be carried out in a relaxed atmosphere and after the elder has become familiar with the provider and more relaxed in the environment.

Remember that most cognitive assessment tools have been developed based on younger adults' responses. The norms for the aged may be quite different.

Do as much as possible to retain comfortable rituals and patterns when assessing and dealing with the aged.

Kane and Kane (1981) Gallo et al. (1988) and Dye (1985) have written excellent texts on assessing the elderly. While the various instruments and methodologies discussed in these texts cannot be dealt with adequately in this chapter, the reader is referred to them for particular techniques.

Importance of Life Experience

In order to assess an aged person humanistically and holistically, one must understand something of the individual's past. Assessments and nursing plans lacking this will reflect a mechanical and often unsuitable model of care. For instance:

When an old lady who taught fourth graders during her working years does serial sevens with alacrity but cannot remember who is president you will understand that discrepancy in abilities.

When an old man berates the nurse, cursing and yelling, it is important to know whether this is a life-long pattern of response to frustration or a newly acquired mode of action that may indicate a brain disorder.

When a lady who has always felt insecure and as if she has been cheated by life accuses the home health aide of stealing from her it is important not to make a quick judgment without knowledge of background and insecurity.

When an old man is provocative sexually it is important to know that sexuality has always been important in his self-concept and assurance of masculinity.

Communication to Gain Understanding

The first consideration in developing an appropriate assessment is to establish *trust* and *rapport*. Below are suggestions that provide guidelines to develop such an assessment.

ESTABLISHING RAPPORT

1. Encourage the individual to ventilate concerns.
2. Listen to hypochondriacal complaints; these need to be expressed.
3. Use touch and active listening skills.
4. Be reliable and dependable; don't promise to do something you can't.
5. Apply therapeutic communication skills.
6. Be cognizant of sensory deficits and adapt an approach to facilitate understanding.
7. Use silence; older persons need time to respond.
8. Address by name person prefers.
9. Respect the "curmudgeon." This conveys coping strength.
10. Encourage reminiscing. When discussing memories, the content and affect is diagnostically significant.
11. Promote autonomy by seeking opinions and giving choices.

Communication forms the basis of data gathering while simultaneously being the foremost mode of intervention. What the caregiver says and does when caring for the aged client provides him or her with a sense of worth or insignificance. Much of this, however, depends on the subtleties of the caregiver's interactions and demonstrations of caring.

Functional Assessment

Level of function is often predictive of the degree of independence and autonomy an aged individual can expect. Most of the aged have three or four chronic diseases but their "wellness" depends on how able they are to negotiate or manage the activities of daily living (ADL). Given the importance of functional status, the assessment must be made in a most discriminating manner. Nursing care emphasis is on improving function, preventing complications, delaying deterioration, facilitating comfort, and in preparing for and providing a dignified death (Wells, 1982). The most useful assessments will underscore needs that must be met in order to achieve these goals rather than become simply a recitation of deficits (Martens, 1986). In addition, nurses are particularly important in assessing functional status. Due to the basic care activities with which they are involved, they are the ones most likely to have a thorough knowledge of the aged client.

Many functional assessment tools already are in use. Most home health and social service agencies have developed their own tools for purposes of case management. Some states have even instituted the use of a single comprehensive assessment instrument that allows for consistency and continuity of care between agencies within the state system. Falcone (1983) has devised a long-term care information system (LTCIS) that has been adopted by several states and is useful in prognostication of intensity of need and specifics for provision of future functional assistance. It would be wise to review this or similar instruments when assessing clients who are likely to need long-term care.

Behavioral Assessment

Socially unacceptable behaviors and acting out of suppressed feelings may trigger an almost automatic assumption of dementia. Incidences may be taken out of context or there may be insufficient attention paid to the precipitants of the behavior within the individual's personal or social system. When assessing the meaning underlying strange behaviors, consider the pointers included below.

FACTORS INFLUENCING BEHAVIOR

When assessing stressors that may underlie erratic behavior, it is important to consider chronic depletion from ongoing illness or deprivation as well as specific traumatic events.

While there is no specific research to confirm the necessity of surveying a particular time span, it may be wise to discuss events of at least the prior two years.

Anger and sometimes aggression are a result of being misinformed or being told half-truths. Caregivers may withhold unpleasant information in an attempt to be kind but it is not uncommon for the aged to "act out" following discovery that they have been misled.

Awareness of an individual's life style and values will often shed light on events that, at first glance, seem behavioral aberrations.

To achieve greater accuracy in methods of observation and documentation of specific behavior patterns, Verstraten (1987) developed a psychogeriatric behavior observation scale. The 14 subscales Verstraten devised offer an interesting delineation that may be used in certain settings to more accurately define problem behaviors. These subscales are divided as follows:

Nonsocial behavior.
Apathetic behavior.
Distorted consciousness.
Loss of decorum.
Rebellious behavior.
Incoherent behavior.
Distorted memory.
Disoriented behavior.
Senseless repetitive behavior.
Restless behavior.
Suspicious behavior.
Melancholy or sorrowful behavior.
Dependent behavior.
Anxious behavior.

It is important to note that such discriminations provide specific information while avoiding judgmental connotations.

Mental Status Assessment

There are several important issues regarding the effectiveness of assessing mental capacity or functional ability of elders. Of most significance is the manner in which the exam results are used. It has been observed that mental status is most usually called into question when the decision of an elder opposes that of family or professionals. It is also known that the evaluative milieu has great impact on achieved results of the test. Therefore, it behooves evaluators to be aware of preconceived notions and expectations of self and others that may influence the validity of test results. The evaluator's personality or attitude inevitably influences his or her perception of others and his or her bias regarding tests of judgment, insight, and conceptual skills. The competency of the evaluator is an issue rarely addressed.

Currently, the imprecision of the various mental status exams leads to frequent difficulty in trying to differentiate dementias from profound depression or intense deprivation. It is also clear that these tests may not reflect whether or not an elderly person is capable of functioning within the social system desired.

Assessment of Physical/Psychiatric Problems

In aged persons, the assessment of a psychiatric problem is most often intermeshed with physical problems. There are rarely the clear lines of demarcation between functional and organic that can be found in younger clients. For this reason, the nurse must become a detective-advocate for thorough medical, psychiatric, and nursing assessment when a disruptive behavioral or emotional disorder is apparent in the client.

In particular, the assessment of dementia must be made with great caution. In an ageist society, consistent feedback of incompetence or ineptitude will often become a self-fulfilling prophecy that is manifest in increasing incompetence, apathy, and withdrawal. What appears to be a vegetative dementia may, in fact, be the progressive debilitation resulting from internalization of negative messages and continual erosion of self-concept. Assessment, therefore, must proceed with care and clarity of all issues involved.

CONCLUSION

This chapter has focused on present issues and concerns underlying the provision of adequate care for the psychogeriatric client: the dearth of qualified professionals, the inappropriate placement in nursing homes of those aged needing mental health services, some emerg-

ing care models, development of more adequately prepared professionals and paraprofessionals, and a brief exposure to issues of assessing the elderly. While progress is occurring, actual needs will not be
met adequately until consumer demands persuade national policy
makers that mental health is as important a priority for our aged as
medical care.

2

Concepts Underlying Care
of the Psychogeriatric Client

This chapter introduces concepts that form the substrate of psychogeriatric care. Knowledge of these is critical to the provision of appropriate care. Stressors and individual coping capacities, self-esteem and self-concept, adequacy of human need fulfillment, sensory changes and particular phase of life problems, such as bereavement, relocation, and retirement are fundamental to understanding the experience of the aged in whatever setting they are encountered.

STRESSORS IN LATE LIFE

Many theorists have addressed the stressors of late life, such as loss of relationships, freedom, finances, health, and possessions. In addition, threats of things to come in the future create a chronic stress: "How will I die?" "Will anyone care when I go?" "Who will care for me if I become unable to care for myself?" "Will I have the ability and capacity to end my life if it becomes unbearable?" These are issues the young and healthy rarely confront. Cowling (1986) found that the major concerns of aging men were health, retirement, dependency, and sexuality. Discussing them with the aged may be useful in assisting them to sort out options. Often, the subjects must be introduced and approached directly as the aged tend to be stoic and self-contained about important issues in their lives. For example, it is common for the aged to focus only on the small uncertainties and discomforts they face each day; but this may be their only way of alerting the caregiver to the disconcerting questions they are constantly asking themselves.

In this regard, Wolanin and Phillips (1981, p. 273) have provided a humanistic and sensitive examination of the potential stressors in both long-term and short-term care settings. Included in their examination are these concerns:

Threats to life and health:
  Apprehension about disability, outcome of illness, and death.
Discomforts:
  Physical problems related to pain, cold, fatigue, unpalatable food, and lack of care.
Loss of a means of subsistence:
  Economic conditions in general and specific to self, significant others, and cost of illness.
Deprivation of intimacy:
  Lack of physical closeness, sexual satisfaction, close affiliations, and friendships.
Enforced idleness:
  Concern about performing usual tasks, engaging in necessary tasks of survival, and engaging in recreational activities.
Restriction of movement:
  Physical immobility, monotony of daily encounters, and absence of personal privacy.
Isolation:
  Separation from usual environment, friends and acquaintances, and perceiving caregivers as uncaring.
Threats to family structure:
  Fear of loss of status/role and concern for failing health and loss of resources of significant others.
Capricious behavior of those in charge:
  Unpredictability of caregivers.
Propaganda:
  Incorrect or incomplete information, withholding of information, and being coerced into something one does not want to do or does not believe.

Awareness of personal degeneration:
Awareness of physical and mental failings and decline.
Rejection:
Feelings of being forgotten, of significant others not caring, and
perceiving the ridicule or dislike of others.
Unknown duration:
Feelings that the confinement will never end and that time drags.
(Wolanin & Phillips, 1981, 273)

Many of these stressors seem specific to aged persons because of the
increasing frequency with which they are hospitalized, their increasing
vulnerability and frailty in late life, and general ageist attitudes they
must confront within themselves and in society at large.

The Wolanin and Phillips (1981) text, however, certainly was not the
first to focus on stressors in late life. Burnside (1973) alerted nurses to
many of the stressors aged persons experience. Twenty years ago, a
series of classic articles appeared in the *Journal of Psychosomatic Research*.
These articles were generated by the group of researchers who developed the "Social Readjustment Rating Scale," more commonly thought
of as the "stress scale" (Holmes & Rahe, 1967). The seminal significance of those pioneering articles was in their efforts to bring some
order and predictive strategies to play on the apparently haphazard and
chaotic events of life. They had already established a relationship between social stressors and illness onset. The major areas of dynamic
significance included changes in family constellation, intimate relationships, occupation, economics, residence, group and peer relationships,
education, religion, recreation, and health. Each life event, to be considered potentially detrimental, required a significant change in the ongoing life pattern of the individual. However, less attention has been paid
to two other significant aspects of this series of studies: the Seriousness
of Illness Rating Scale (Wyler, Masuda, & Holmes, 1968) and Quantitative Study of Recall of Life Events (Casey, Masuda, & Holmes,
1967). It appears that, in ranking, the seriousness of illness, impairment
of function is viewed as thoughtfully as threat to life in many instances.
The other important finding was that consistency of recall of life events
was directly related to the importance the individual attributed to them.
Unfortunately, there was no subgroup of respondents to this study that
were over 65 years of age. To account for this lacuna in the research
base, nurses should investigate the ranking and recall validity of illness
experiences by very old clients. The recently devised Stokes-Gordon
Stress Scale (1988) is designed specifically to evaluate the stressors of
elders (see Appendix).

Stress Reactions

By far the most common stress in the lives of elders is illness or the threat of illness, which usually gives rise to thoughts about mortality. Illness may also precipitate loss of self-trust, changes in self-concept, alteration in interpersonal relationships, and fears of permanent dependency. Thus, illness often heralds the development of depression, anxiety reactions, paranoid responses, or other psychiatric disturbances (Sakayue, 1986). Within an institutional setting, such problems may increase in severity and frequency due to limitations in psychosocial supports, cognitive limitations, and suppressed coping styles. External factors, such as acuity of illness, life-style discontinuity, attitudes of significant others, and social network supports will also influence the patient's response.

Knowledge of the premorbid personality style of the patient may be useful in selecting therapeutic interventions. Graves and Kucharski (1978) elaborated on typical reactions to illness of three personality types (obsessional, hysterical, and narcissistic). They found that the obsessional personality may be more typical of the elderly when illness is perceived as loss of control or punishment for not taking sufficient care of oneself in the past. Such types are problem solvers by nature but often bog down in rumination without reaching decisions. There is considerable therapeutic value in engaging them in mutual problem exploration, providing detailed information about the issues and focusing on making meaningful connections between thoughts and their emotional impact.

The hysterical personalities tend to become less dramatic in their later years but still enjoy precipitating reactions to their behavior. These persons need to be recognized and acknowledged for dramatizations that are not detrimental. The narcissistic person may become more self-absorbed in the process of aging. It is useful to employ this tendency in therapeutic ways such as keeping a journal of thoughts and feelings, a dream diary or a health diary. These can be legitimized by professionals as valuable sources of information while they provide the egocentric person with an outlet that is productive.

Because there are multiple problems to solve related to stress reactions in the elderly, the creative capacities of caregivers, family, and clients will be strained. Knowing this, it may be encouraging to remember that interventions which bring about positive results in any way will have ramifications for all other problems and may even prevent a "negative outcome" (Engel, 1980).

There are several common psychosocial problems of aging that must be considered in assessing an individual's stressors and adaptive level of function. Table 2.1 presents these problems and possible reactions to them.

While these stressors do not necessarily result in emotional disorders, even "survivors" may find coping energies greatly reduced in their presence. Therefore, their appearance requires that the caregiver consider appropriate counteractive interventions.

DSM III-R Classifications of Stressors

The Diagnostic Statistical Manual, 3rd Revision (DSM III-R) provides detailed information for categorizing psychiatric and emotional disorders. The diagnoses derived from the DSM III-R provide a national data base for determining frequency of various mental and emotional disorders. In the DSM III Revision distinctions have been made that provide a more realistic and useful diagnosis of some problems of the aged.

In response to the DSM III Revisions, Axis IV distinctions between acute and enduring stressors have significant implications in diagnos-

TABLE 2.1 Stressors in Late Life

Pain and chronic discomfort	Arthritis
Sensory loss	Normal aging changes
Translocation crises	Hospitalizations
	Protective settings
	Moving in with children
	Insufficient income
Loneliness and grief	Loss of significant others
	Isolation
	Disengagement
	Chronic bereavement
Sexual frustration	Lack of partner
	Imbalance of the sexes
	Aging changes
	Incompatibility
	Ageist messages
	Depression
Meaninglessness	Anomie
	Social exclusion
	Social irrelevance
	Not being needed
Family problems	Dependency
	Abuse
	Favoritism
	Incompatibility
	Role reversal

ing problems of the aged. Because acute stressors will produce crisis symptomatology and enduring stressors will markedly lower the coping energies available to the individual, the clinician must discriminate accurately between them. See Table 2.2 below for the likely types of which to be aware.

Axis V includes current level of overall adaptive functioning as well as the highest level in the past year. In assessing the aged, the discrimination is significant and intrinsically tied to the stressors experienced. The onset of psychiatric symptomatology often correlates with stress overload, even among those who have had a pattern of mental disturbance for some time.

SELF-ESTEEM AND SELF-CONCEPT

Self-esteem is the opinion one holds of self and the judgment inherent in that opinion. High self-esteem is based on feelings of effectiveness, good role performance, the opinions of one that others hold, ability to positively influence those one cares about, and all the components of self-concept that are congruent with the particular cultural or social ideal.

Much has been said about ageist attitudes and the effects this may have on elders' self-esteem. Yet the collective ageist attitude has little to do with how an individual feels about self as older persons rarely identify with the aged until they are ill or functionally incompetent. When one is effective in executing socially respected roles or has attained a powerful position in society, one seems able to maintain self-esteem into late old age. Unfortunately, the tendency of optimists to focus on the successes of the remarkable old may further decrease self-esteem of elders with some impairments. In this respect, what can caregivers do to increase self-esteem of the functionally impaired older individual? Developing meaningful social roles and respectful

TABLE 2.2 DSM III-R Classification of Stressors

Acute	Enduring
Relocation	Alterations in sensory function
Losses	Alterations in role performance
Abuse	Neglect
Acute illness	Chronic illness
	Alterations in self care
	Alterations in sexuality

social interactions, ensuring the opportunity to participate in enriching events, and making visible the impact of the aged on society in the present and the past are all viable options. It must be remembered that their toil and tenacity has made possible the progress our nation has experienced. Caregivers must let them know they recognize this debt, individually and collectively, and will "reimburse" with sensitivity, intelligence, and compassion.

Self-esteem is one of the hallmarks of mental health. It develops slowly as an adolescent establishes an adult identity and the components of self-concept become clear and satisfying. Other major components of self-concept include perceived identity, role functions, sexual identity, talents and abilities, territorial influence, appearance, and attitudes toward self. In any of these arenas, interventions can be planned to maintain or enhance self-esteem.

Maintenance of self-concept and self-esteem are critical to coherent behavior. Yet they are difficult to accomplish in institutional settings designed more for the efficiency of facility function than intimate patient care. While most settings have made genuine efforts to become more efficient, they have also lost sight of the individual patient. A check list may be useful to confirm that individualized approaches of concrete nature have been implemented. The following may provide guidelines to which facilities may add their specific ideas and actions:

Each resident's photograph is included in chart.
Each resident's photograph is posted on door of room.
Photographs of significant people are in the room.
Select furnishings have been brought in by resident.
Staff are aware of resident's previous occupation.
Staff know something of resident's life history.
Specific strengths of resident have been identified and are being used.
Each resident has one particular ally on staff who coordinates care.
Each resident is involved in one small group selected with their particular needs in mind.
Each resident has short-term goals he or she is motivated to work toward.

Upon admission to a facility, many of these actions can be immediately implemented. An effective way of getting to know patients and their needs is to begin with the "name game." This has been particularly useful in getting acquainted and providing assurance that each resident is significant and that staff are interested in them as individuals. To play the "name game," you can begin with staff. They will enjoy it fully as much as a group of patients.

While the rules are simple, the effect may be, as mentioned above, more than beneficial. Each individual gives his or her full name and tells all he or she knows about its origin, meaning, who chose it, nicknames, and whether or not he or she likes the name. What does the name mean in terms of self-definition? The added advantage of doing this exercise is to assist others to remember the individual's name. Given the significance and importance we each attach to our name, it is certainly worth the time to focus on this aspect of self-concept. As a result, some women have even gotten into discussions of maiden name, marriage, and women's issues as they discuss changing their surname when married.

Another nursing tool in definition of self-concept is the camera. Stotts and Pickett (1987) report on the extensive use of cameras in nursing situations. For our purposes, they suggest using photos on bulletin boards to feature certain residents and their life histories or specific accomplishments. Many facilities have instituted similar uses of resident photographs, all to good effect.

Residents seem to respond to being photographed by increased interest in appearance and grooming, recovering a sense of personal significance, and enjoyment of the attention. In addition, photographs can graphically demonstrate "before and after" effects, such as changes in posture, weight loss or gain, and improved grooming. It would be useful if photographs of long-term patients were taken routinely and periodically and kept in the chart to show changes over time.

Staff seem to take greater interest in residents as they photograph them and plan for their individual needs based upon more careful observation. Some become quite involved in the artistry of their photographs and go on to more extensive photography projects such as creating facility albums or giving photographic presentations at professional meetings. Some, such as Rod Schmall and Marianne Gontarz, have gained national recognition for their sensitive photographic portrayals of the aged (American Society on Aging, Photographic Essay Displays and Awards, 1982 through 1989).

Like the camera, video recording is also a useful tool for defining self-concept, particularly because it can feature an action in progress. Residents often respond positively to being shot or to shooting themselves. As one resident said, "This is just like being in the movies." I have not found reports of situations in which residents have been videotaped when actually performing, or in skits and dramas. There seems to be much potential in such activities.

Belongings as Elements of Self-Concept

As one grows older and gathers possessions, one begins to conceive of them as extensions of one's being, embodying something of the events and people involved in their accumulation. As such, they become part of a person's self-concept and personal security. As Margaret Mead so astutely wrote in *Blackberry Winter* (1972), she took her special paper-weight wherever she went. No matter how different the culture she visited, this kept her oriented to self and security. In this respect, one factor in relocation adjustment of elders is whether or not they are able to take cherished possessions with them.

McCracken (1987) surveyed the emotional impact of possession loss on widows relocated to small, low-rent housing units. She found that the most important possessions moved were, in rank order:

Bedroom furniture
Television
Photographs

The items that could not be moved and were most missed were, in rank order:

Appliances
Baking utensils
Pets
Garden tools

The individuals expressed the loss of possessions as a loss of personal history and sense of self. While these individuals were still living in the community and managing their lives quite independently, caregivers may extrapolate their feelings, if not the importance of specific items, to the institutionalized or hospitalized persons we serve. It would seem imperative that every individual in any unfamiliar setting has at least one item of choice that affirms identity and sustains self-concept. This seems a relatively simple intervention to plan and activate.

Cultural and Generational Differences in Self-Concept

Elderly persons are often of a unique cultural heritage, perhaps one generation from the "Old Country." In late life, they may have an overwhelming desire to return or to speak the mother language with someone who understands simply in order to strengthen their sense of

self. To help them return, if only in memory or with pictorial jour-
neys, preserves a sense of self-identity and meaning. In a multicultural
society such as ours, we must be cognizant of tradition and culture. To
illustrate this, Figure 2.1 identifies specific cultural needs.

The elements illustrated in Figure 2.1 show the various fundamental beliefs, life patterns and structures, and even dietary preferences
that may influence self-concept. Unless we are cognizant of these
many factors we cannot hope to understand how to meet the needs of
clients.

Nursing Diagnoses Related to Self-Esteem and Self-Concept

As defined by Murray (1984), *self-concept* describes the totality of
one's perception of self and includes elements of multiple, ever changing components of one's life experience. Ordinarily, self-concept is
rooted in coping skills and changes gradually as one matures. During

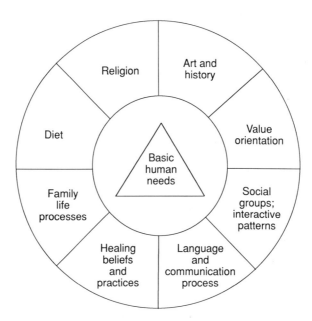

Figure 2.1   Components of Orque's Ethnic-Cultural Systemic Framework

(Modified from Orque, M., Block, B., and Monroy, L.: 1983. Ethnic nursing care: a multicul-
tural approach, The C.V. Mosby Co., St. Louis.)
From Ebersole, P., & Hess, P. (1985). *Toward Healthy Aging: Human Needs and Nursing
Response*, 2nd ed. St. Louis: C. V. Mosby.

crisis situations, however, and in certain mental disorders, self-concept can undergo serious disturbance. Disturbance in self-concept may be related to the following psychiatric conditions:

organic mental syndromes (usually in the early phases);
mood disorders;
somatoform disorders; and
gender and sexual disorders.

To further define the components of self-concept, refer to the list below.

COMPONENTS OF SELF-CONCEPT

Reactions of others to behavior and appearance from infancy throughout life.
Norms of the culture, socioeconomic strata, religion, and age norms not mentioned by Murray (1984) are especially important.
Family norms, relationships, values, size, and birth order.
Interpretations of other's reactions to self.
Attempts at class mobility.
Geographic history.
Physical appearance and function, including sex, age, and sensory motor perceptions.
Physical, emotional, and social developmental stages of self.
Attitudes and emotions regarding body parts considered strategically important, such as nose, skin, hair, and sex organs.
Internal drives, dependency needs, and ideals to which one aspires.
Identification of others who are considered as role models.
Roles, occupation, and various activities in which one is involved.
Unity of memory, on which one's continuity of self is based.
(Murray, 1984)

Nursing diagnoses related to disturbance in self-concept may include:

Ineffective individual coping
Anxiety

Fear
Isolation

In all cases, to intervene effectively it is important to identify the components of self-concept that are perceived by the individual to be threatened, unacceptable, or devalued. Similarly, it is important to identify those components of self-concept that express strength and more positive, adaptive behavior (Martens, 1986).

Nursing Care Plan for Negative Self-Concept

Murray (1984) has constructed a nursing care plan using negative self-concept as a model for mental health nurses, which is particularly relevant for geropsychiatric nurses. By the time one is old, of course, the formative aspects of self-concept are deeply embedded in the personality. However, more ubiquitous in late life are stressors that erode the self-concept, which can give rise to particularly conflictive situations heretofore unexperienced by the aged person.

It is important to remember that the factors that most influence self-concept are within the expected norms of culture, sex, family, role, developmental stage, and appearance. Self-concept also is largely derived from feedback. In the later years, the accumulation of memories either reinforces continuity and acceptability of self or erodes one's self-esteem. However, because self-concept is so responsive to consistent positive input from respected others, it is subject to modification in a healing manner. Through the therapeutic relationship, then, the geropsychiatric nurse is in an excellent position to modify self-concept. To accomplish this, Murray (1985) articulated short-term goals and outcome criteria for ready adaptation to many client situations. Table 2.3 illustrates Murray's design.

In an ageist society, rebuilding a positive self-concept has become a frequent goal for the older population.

THE HIERARCHY OF HUMAN NEEDS

While a conceptual framework modeled after human need is not the organizational pattern of this book, human need does provide a simplified way of ordering priorities and understanding a client's major focus of concern. In general, human need must be addressed in a hierarchical manner. Maslow's (1970) concept of human need includes:

TABLE 2.3 Model Nursing Care Plan — Self-Concept

Data	NSG diagnosis	Outcome criteria	Interventions	Evaluation
Subjective data: "I have always prided myself on not asking anything from anybody." Objective data: Client manages own home nicely. Client is well groomed. Client takes care of her garden. Client cares for grandchild and refuses to accept anything for her effort.	Potential disturbance in self-concept related to the possibility of needing assistance.	Client will accept money for care of grandchild. Client will discuss a plan for assistance with house and garden chores. Client will express feelings about maintaining her independence. Client will allow me to help her fix lunch. Client will treat herself to a massage.	Encourage client to call agencies that provide services for elders so that she will be prepared if she needs help. Discuss the enjoyment family may derive from helping her at times. Encourage client to talk about her fears of future frailty. Explore client's feelings about letting others help her. Offer to assist client in preparing lunch. Discuss massage and provide phone number of masseuse.	Client called Senior Service Agency to identify sources of help if she needs it. Client unwilling to accept money for care of grandchild but will allow children to do some of the heavy chores in home and garden. Client spoke of feeling that others would be annoyed if she asked them for help. Client allowed me to bring snack to share at our next meeting. Client rejected idea of a massage. She felt that would be "pampering" herself.

37

- Maintenance of basic biologic integrity through provisions for food, rest, shelter, and organ function.
- Seeking safety and personal security in an environment designed for personal comfort and function.
- Development and cultivation of a self-system that provides assurance of a sense of belonging.
- Finding opportunities to express self toward ego enhancement and mastery.
- Seeking meaning and purpose beyond one's individual needs and desires.

This hierarchy forms a useful basis for organizing efforts to provide a milieu for survival and personal growth. Figure 2.2 illustrates a useful synopsis of particular needs, symptoms of need deprivation, and suggested interventions responsive to the need.

In addition, there are certain general guidelines for intervention with elderly persons (provided below) that will be useful in most cases.

GENERAL GUIDELINES FOR INTERVENTION

1. Be active and direct in interactions.
2. Recognize and promote individuality.
3. Do not patronize.
4. Plan activities that give opportunities for success.
5. Encourage and assist if necessary in good grooming.
6. Involve client in assisting others. The need to be needed is extremely important.
7. Accept the validity of the client's feelings.
8. Project an optimistic attitude.
9. Share something of yourself and let them know what you learn from them.

Unmet Needs

Elders with mental health problems are, like everyone else, in need of self-respect, friendship, affection, mental stimulation, some sense of achievement, and a sense of safety and security in addition to physical care. The complexity of assisting patients to achieve the maximum level of life satisfaction and self-actualization is related to the unique and long life history the patient brings to the situation. Good care demands recognition of the patient's unique perspective. Satisfactory physical care is designed to help the individual function in order to

Problems	Symptoms	(Maslow level)	Needs	Interventions
Social clocks Self-fulfilling prophesies Routinized life	Apathy Rigidity Boredom Ennui	Self-Actualization	Self-expression New situations Self-transcendence Stimulation	Creative pursuits Meditation Reflection Fantasy Teaching/learning Relaxation
Social devaluation Lack of Role Meaninglessness Little autonomy	Delusions Paranoia Depression Anger Indecisive	Self-esteem	Control Success To be needed	Reminiscing Control of money Activate latent interests Allowed to help others Identify legacy
Displacement Losses	Depression Hallucinations Alienation Loneliness	Belonging	Territory Friends Family Group affiliation Philosophy Confidante	Significant objects Pets, plants Soap opera families Touch group participation Listening Fictive kin
Sensory losses Limited mobility Translocation	Illusions Hallucinations Confusion Compulsions Obsessions Fear/anxiety	Safety and security	Safe environment Sensory accoutrements Mobility	Familiar routines Spaced stimulation Explanations Environmental cues
Homeostatic resilience Poor nutrition Medications Income Subclinical diseases (Birren) Pain	Confusion Depression Fear Anxiety Disorientation	Biologic integrity	Food Shelter Sex Rest Body Integrity Comfort	Adequate resources Knowledge of medications Conservation of energy Napping Small, frequent meals Choices of food

Figure 2.2 Nursing Process and Maslow's Hierarchy of Needs

Reprinted with permission. From A. Maslow, *Motivation and Personality* (2nd ed.) © 1970. Harper & Row.

find meaning and purpose in living. When psychosocial needs are ignored or unmet, these needs may be expressed in oblique and unusual ways. Figure 2.3 illustrates the complexity of this situation. *Acting out behaviors* is the term typically used to describe difficult behaviors of persons who do not express their feelings and needs more directly. The aged may be more likely to engage in them if there seems to be no one expressing interest in their inner world of feelings and suppressed needs. Common examples of acting out behaviors for the aged include overt and inappropriate expression of sexual feelings. If there are no appropriate avenues of expression or no one gives

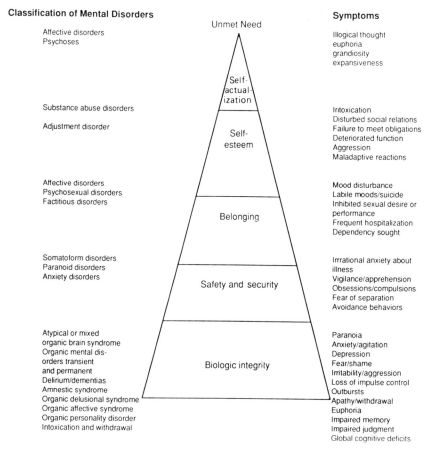

Figure 2.3   Mental disorders Related to Unmet Needs

Source: From P. Ebersole & P. Hess. (1985). *Toward Healthy Aging: Human Needs and Nursing Response*, 2nd Ed. St. Louis; C. V. Mosby.

credence to the validity of sexual feelings in late life, then the individual may become blatant about sexually provocative behaviors. Likewise, aggression often is a means of expressing anger at waning capacities. In addition, aging itself and its assaults on life may be rejected, which can lead to even more serious consequences. In this regard, suicide can be seen as a dynamic, if desperate, acting out of a statement of self-assertion that emphasizes an ability to take charge and direct the course of one's life—even if that course is toward death. Nonparticipation can also be a subtle means of declaring one's right to decide.

In general, each behavior can be seen as a statement of need. Recognizing the implicit statement is the key to management of troublesome behaviors. Approaching the desired change in behavior directly can be fruitful if the individual is also given recognition for the feelings that underlie the statement of need.

Cuizon-Saiz (personal communication, 1988) provides a particularly illustrative example of a patient with unmet needs.

Mrs. L. was a shrewd and difficult lady to care for. She particularly rebelled against taking a shower. She began to alienate the staff by her abusive and hostile reaction when they attempted to get her to shower. One nursing assistant said she was "the fastest shower giver in the West." This provocative approach stimulated interest in Mrs. L. who was in need of someone to challenge. She remonstrated that she got exceedingly cold when showering. A quick, warm shower followed immediately by a warm blanket was well tolerated by Mrs. L. even though she complained throughout the procedure. Further insight into Mrs. L.'s personality demonstrated that she liked to challenge and test others but became irate when treated mechanically. When the staff joked or challenged her, she responded well.

Noncompliance is a judgmental and often inappropriate means of describing an individual's behavior. It assumes that the health care provider is correct in the requests made of the patient and that the patient is recalcitrant or openly rebellious in following a therapeutic regimen. However, ignoring treatment plans may be one of the only ways open to the patient to express autonomy and decision-making capacity. It is incumbent on the provider to determine if the patient has sufficient information about the treatment plan to make an informed judgment related to following the directives and if he or she understands the consequences of noncompliance.

According to Hussian (1986), often medication is the issue of noncompliance. Unless the noncompliance is life threatening or seriously disruptive to the environment, the patient must be given the option of not following the treatment plan. When failure to conform is purely due to poor memory or inattention, it may be useful to employ discriminative stimuli. For example, in a conspicuous place tape a brightly colored chart depicting a specific activity required at a particular time. The chart could feature a picture of the medication beside a plate of food to remind the patient to take the medication at mealtimes. Compliance may also be encouraged by affiliation with another individual participating in a similar treatment program or activity. Group reinforcement has been found helpful.

Opportunities to participate in activities consistent with personal talents, values, and interests provide an occasion for both decisional and behavioral control. Talents may be as varied as playing the piano, gardening, reading mail to others, or finding an influential voice.

Again, Cuizon-Saiz (1988) provides an example of a patient who benefited from an opportunity to participate.

> Mrs. T. was a lady of 80 years with a Jewish background who had experienced Hitler's Germany. She had escaped through China to the United States. Given her background and oppressive past, she became loud and obtrusive in her later years when she developed a mild dementia. When she was admitted to the nursing home, she was immediately labeled as incorrigible. She objected to everything that occurred and, in the activity room, her voice could be heard above all others no matter what was happening. The activity director recognized the need for attention and some element of control. She asked Mrs. T. to become involved in the resident council and encouraged her to accept the office of treasurer. When Mrs. T. realized she had influence and others were respectful of her position, she was able to temper her loud and offensive behaviors. She never expressed her deep feelings or needs.

The need to be needed seems never to be extinguished. To cope with the changes they are experiencing, elders may become more self-absorbed and narcissistic in their concerns. Aside from this propensity toward egocentricity, however, it is also apparent that the ability to actively contribute to the welfare of others is important. Many elders express this by their concern for family, sometimes to the extent of sacrificing themselves. Some say, "My family would like me to live with them but I would be a burden." Whether this is a fact or fantasy, it serves the purpose of helping the elder see some meaning and purpose in a situation he or she may find unbearable.

SENSORY CHANGES THAT AFFECT COPING

Sensory decrements in the aged, both normal and abnormal, have been frequently discussed and much literature addresses the needs

accompanying decreased acuity and ability to attend to environmental cues. I will consider these issues briefly. For more in-depth
discussion of sensory changes, I refer the reader to the Ebersole and
Hess (1990) text, "Toward Healthy Aging: Human Needs and Nursing Response."

As one ages, there is a general decline in acuity of all senses. When
this decline is normal, an individual's life experience largely compen-
sates. Unfortunately, however, a "normal" decline has yet to be
defined, especially when related to the variety of environmental
assaults each individual faces as he or she ages. Notwithstanding
this lack of definition, to enrich the experience of an elderly client,
care plans should include enhancing sensory capacity when possible.

Vision

Visual problems begin sometime in middle age with the flattening of
the visual orb and the need for magnification of close work. Cataracts
usually begin developing in the seventh decade and can be readily
remedied with surgery on an outpatient basis. Yellowing of the eye
lens tends to change the perception of tone and hue of certain colors
and make the surroundings appear more bland. Bright primary colors
may be attractive but not soothing. In this respect, color coordination
should be done with a particular setting in mind. In general, however,
visual deficits categorically seem to have little to do with mental
health of elders.

Hearing

While elders adapt well to most sensory decrements that are gradual
and expected, their mental health often is affected by hearing impairment. Hearing impairment not only is the most frequent and earliest
sensory loss, but it affects human relationships and communication in
profound or subtle ways. One lady told of losing her hearing abruptly
following a bout with encephalitis. She began to understand the term
"deaf and dumb" as she found people treating her as if she could not
think any better than she could hear. Clerks followed her through
stores as if she were dangerous or a shoplifter. Some people acted as if
she did not exist and totally ignored her presence at social gatherings.
Eventually she found a specialized apparatus that can compensate for
some otic nerve damage. Because technology in hearing aid development has progressed so rapidly, individuals who have not previously
found hearing aids satisfactory for them are advised to seek an audiol-
ogy clinic for reassessment and exposure to newer aids that they may

find acceptable. There are many new types of hearing aids on the market and an audiologic clinic will provide opportunity to try most of them. Heaing aid outlets, on the other hand, are limited to the few that they are particularly interested in marketing. In reality, most elders have never had audiometric testing in spite of the prevalence of hearing disorders in the older population. Professionals are advised to discuss hearing with every older individual they serve. In the case of those with emotional disorders, the inability to correctly perceive what others are saying may be a major contributor to anxiety and suspicious feelings.

When working with the hearing impaired in an institution, it is helpful to have some identifying clothing or symbol to alert others to the hearing deficit. Usually, an individual hears out of one ear better than the other, and this hearing preference should be made known to staff and others. If the individual seems to distort messages, it can be useful to ask what he or she heard. One aged man thought a social worker told him he was "cutely dressed" when, in fact, she had told him he appeared to be "acutely distressed."

In general, caregivers must note that all sensory decrements may contribute to a sense of apathy and disinterest in surroundings as well as misinterpretations.

PHASE OF LIFE PROBLEMS

Within the parameters defined by the DSM III-R, those conditions that become a focus of treatment, but are not considered a mental disorder, are Axis V codes. The large range of conditions and situations therein covered include many that are frequent concomitants of aging. Such phase of life problems often include issues of dealing with personal mortality, despair, meaninglessness, and reduced capacities. The most frequent precipitants of these issues include bereavement, relocation, and retirement.

Long-standing marital problems may exist that are exacerbated by the demands, stressors, and reduced capacities of the aged. In addition, parent–child problems may occur as roles and relationships are redefined. Aspects of family history and favoritism long forgotten may emerge. Family members other than spouse and children may also be affected by changes in the family circumstances and interpersonal relationships. Often a niece, nephew, grandchild, or in-law may be extremely significant in the family drama that caregivers must address. Because the family provides the majority of care of elders and the issues are complex, I have devoted Chapter 7 to families as care-givers.

Bereavement

Uncomplicated bereavement is probably the most frequently encoun-tered of all problems with the aged. Losses accumulate with the aging process until in very old age few cohorts are left who can share in a common pool of memories. The loss of spouse must be anticipated but the loss of a child seems to be the most grievous of all. Uncompli-cated bereavement is evidenced by severe depression that is resolved in time. Morbid preoccupation with guilt, feelings of worthlessness that do not abate, and marked functional impairment are indices that the grief pattern is not progressing normally. In late life, it may be difficult to judge the normality of a grief reaction, primarily because the compounded processes of losses overlapping may produce a chronic grief state. Unfortunately, to this date chronic grief patterns have not been adequately studied.

According to Kübler-Ross (in Gill, 1980), every loss is a "small death" and with each we go through a compressed grief process. In this respect, the aged have many "small deaths." Because of the frequency of more serious losses, they may react strongly to what others might consider inconsequential losses. For instance, Mabel was seriously depressed when the birdbath in the back of her house was stolen. Yes, she could buy another birdbath but this one had been handmade by her uncle 30 years before. Nor had she only lost the birdbath, but something more: faith in the neighborhood she had, for so many years, considered safe. As a result, her sense of security vanished. What next would be taken from her?

When working with the aged, bear in mind that the magnitude of the loss as it appears may have no relationship to the impact it will have on the individual. Therefore, it is important to bring the aged person's feelings out into the open. A caregiver might do this by saying, "You recently suffered a loss. How are you managing?" If the elder is not inclined to share feelings when invited to do so, that is perfectly acceptable. However, it is not acceptable for caregivers to ignore the subject simply because it is painful or seems inconsequential.

Each small loss may, in fact, be felt by elders as a chipping away at their defenses against the loss of self, the ultimate loss. For most young adults, it is difficult to perceive this feeling of marking the days toward the last of life. As a result, caregivers should be especially concerned with an elder's "unfinished business," and show constant sensitivity to appreciating the small joys perhaps shared with the elder each day prior to death.

Helping Caregivers Cope with the Dying

For gerontic health care providers, dealing with dying persons is a continual issue. Of course, reactions to the death of elderly patients will vary depending upon the level of attachment and the length of the relationship. Unfortunately, health care providers often brush aside the grief they experience as "unprofessional," which is a mistake. It is important, therefore, to develop a consistent mechanism for staff to deal with the deaths of patients. When these are in place and expected, each individual will be more comfortable in sharing feelings and reactions. Lardaro (1987) suggests a post mortem staff meeting as well as regular meetings to discuss anticipated deaths. Ideally, these meetings should also include other patients who had been close to the deceased as well as available family members. Sharing between professionals, family, and patients would increase the support and understanding as well as give recognition to the significance placed on patients and their lives and deaths.

In addition, health care providers working in settings where death of clients is frequent and expected may need an educational group process to help them understand grief process and grief resolution. Dagon and Van Sickle (1987) constructed such a group for the education of geropsychiatric fellows. The ten-week closed support group focused on education, community resources for the bereaved, expression of previous experiences of loss, and keeping a diary of reactions during the period of attendance. Bereaved elderly were recruited from the community as group participants. This model seems to hold promise for application to many health care professionals.

Grief management by health care providers often presents difficulties because of lack of training. Gordon (1987) suggests the following topics for seminars to assist those who need direction in coping with the dying and their own reactions:

The impact of personal experiences with death on the professional role.
Promotion of patient autonomy at the end of life.
Learning to let go and not feel like a failure.
Appropriate grieving and surviving repeated loss of patients.
Understanding the nonrational elements of dying.

Sensitivity to diverse ethnic, religious, and family traditions that are important at the end of life.

Dealing with Dying

Assisting clients to die at home is becoming a more frequent activity of health care providers and a more expressed desire of patients. Levine (1983) found that four of five people wish to die at home, although, in reality, four of five people die in institutions. When there is a home where a patient may go to die and if that is the wish of that patient, every effort should be made to assist the patient and the family in making it a growth experience. To make dying at home easier, Levine has also suggested the following:

A cassette recorder for the person to listen to selected music and guided meditation tapes.
A bedside bell for the person to summon attention.
Daily baths and gentle massage.
A variety of fluids should always be available.
A hospital bed only if desired; many prefer to die in their own bed.
The bed should be placed near a window, or in the living room where the person can participate in family activities.
The person should have control of his or her own pain medication when at all possible.
Meanings of death and feelings should be discussed openly.
Visiting nurses and hospice services may be helpful.

Relocation Adjustment

Housing and living situations affect adaptation in as yet poorly understood ways. Continuity of care for geropsychiatric patients across a variety of institutional and community-based settings has not been given the attention it deserves. Relocation stress and trauma can be reduced significantly by prior preparation, preservation of autonomy, and followup by persons from the prior setting to assist in problem solving and adjustment to the new setting.

Intra-institutional relocation is an additional stress to individuals already coping with disease, disability, and lack of autonomy. Programs for information and preparation of individuals and their families when a move is necessary may facilitate the adaptation. Introduction to a "patient pal" from the new unit will pave the way and may increase the self-esteem of both patients.

A report from Sweden (Annerstedt, 1987) emphasizes the beneficial results obtained when cognitively impaired elders were relocated from nursing homes or homes to small collectives. Settings housing approximately ten patients were selected. Staff reported increased psychomotor activity, affectual expression, and cognitive function. It was concluded that psychosocial and environmental factors are significant in the adaptation of impaired elders. Given the health care industry and economic priorities in the United States, this model is unlikely to be seriously considered here. However, the concept could be adapted rather easily to long-term care. Some facilities have already designed into care plans provision for a pseudo-family atmosphere and a specific group of patients and staff to which one feels allegiance and a sense of belonging. These efforts might be enhanced to provide "small scale housing" within a large facility. Increases in individualized care, security, and closeness would enhance the quality of life significantly for staff and patients.

In dealing with individuals who are experiencing their first admission to a psychogeriatric ward, it is particularly important to assess life stresses and functional capacity prior to emergence of significant problems. Most commonly, a major loss is precedent to first admission. While most of these patients have lived independently, often they are discharged to nursing homes. Symptomatology or diagnosis alone is insufficient to determine the need for a protected setting. These determinations should be made with great caution and sensitivity to the self-concept implications previously discussed.

Facilitating Institutional Adjustment   Institutions exist to serve the needs of patients yet there is limited tolerance for needs they are not prepared to meet. Of necessity, the patient must comply with certain routines and rules of the institution to ensure the maintenance of the milieu and respect for the rights of all patients. Patients vary in their ability to do so, however. Each individual's rights and privileges must be negotiated with these things in mind.

Many patient problems may arise from institutionalization. No one has yet provided clear insights into all the ramifications of leaving a community life style, where freedom of choice prevails, to a life where such freedom is severely retricted. While transfer to an institution is often necessary, this does not make it any more acceptable to the individual being transferred. However, if the environment was altered to more closely resemble a normal living situation, individual problems arising from transfer might not emerge or fulminate. Schafer (1985) has identified 11 approaches that may modify the environment to more nearly resemble one's previous living situation:

Individualize care.
Learn who the patient is.
Recognize strengths.
Foster sense of control.
Provide environmental cues for orientation.
Maintain patient's home schedule.
Adapt schedule of diagnostic procedures to patient's needs.
Communicate.
Time the giving of information.
Maintain consistency in staff–patient interactions.
Maintain ADL using patient's coping resources and social supports.

All these suggestions require re-thinking of the way care is usually provided in long-term institutions. Recognizing the limitation of personnel and resources in such situations, health care providers must be creative. What then are the practical and possible ways these suggestions might be achieved?

Individualized care might begin with a psychosocial admission assessment that would include data about the client's preferences, home schedules, strengths, and ability to accomplish ADLs before admission to the facility. This will require additional time during the admission process and will probably include information from the family as well as the patient. Making the additional effort to do this would undoubtedly save time later in the reduction of patient problem behaviors and by keeping the family vitally involved in patient care. If this is done well, several of the other suggestions will already have been implemented. Gaining data on the life history of the patient can be interesting and rewarding as the "patient" begins to become a "person" in the minds of the staff. Ideally, the staff who works most with that individual will be assigned to obtain a life history of significant roles, life events, and activities that have given the individual his or her sense of identity.

When adequate data has been obtained, it should be discussed or readily accessible to the caregiving team. In this way, advance planning regarding schedules and preferences can be initiated and evaluated. When trying to imagine the effects of this individualization on staff, meal, and activity schedules, it may seem formidable. However, if each patient is approached in this manner, patterns would emerge and staffing might be shifted to accommodate. For instance, those who preferred a late evening meal could simply have it prepared in advance and ready for microwave at their preferred time. For those who preferred an evening bath to a morning shower, the family might be enlisted to help. Often, the family would be relieved to have a concrete task to perform.

Consistency in staff–patient interactions has two components: consistency of staff and consistency of interactions. Staff consistency can be difficult but each patient can be assigned to a particular staff who they know is their advocate and who, in turn, knows them well. When primary care nursing is not always possible, modified primary care can be implemented. Clear communication in terms of expectations, restrictions, and areas where one has choice could be the responsibility of the primary staff, however. It is important the individual can identify a primary staff ally to facilitate institutional adjustment.

Retirement Adjustment

Any situation that disturbs the nature or satisfaction of the relationship network, whether primary or secondary, is likely to result in social isolation. Below are listed psychiatric diagnoses that may precipitate social isolation:

Organic mental syndromes
Delusional paranoid disorders
Mood disorders
Adjustment disorders
Bereavement
Phase of life or life circumstance problems

Social isolation related to retirement adjustment (phase of life problems) and concomitant income reduction, is considered below as an exemplifying condition.

Clearly, in many assessments this diagnosis would be overlooked unless the nurse is alert to the individual's life style and maintains a holistic approach to caregiving. Gerontologic literature notes that the transitional year of retirement is significant and predictive of the positive or negative nature of the retirement adjustment. No longer is it held true that retirement itself produces illness, decline, and death. If the nurse takes a careful social history of his or her client, it becomes clear if the client has sought out social contacts and activities or whether he or she has relied on those "ready-made" in relation to profession or job. In those cases, a potential problem related to retirement adjustment will usually appear as depression, isolation, and illness. In addition, there would likely be a corollary nursing diagnosis of disturbance in self-concept related to retirement. Because both diagnoses would require interventions specific to successful resolution of each, nurses would need to identify them individually. Planned intervention in avoiding social isolation would include anticipatory guidance prior to actual retirement; in effect, a gradual weaning from job-related social activities to other retirement-related activities. In this respect, the nurse is usually seen as one who can suggest appropriate resources and activities and act as a sounding board for unexpected feelings and reactions which may occur. Major interventions in the same situation but in response to the nursing diagnosis "disturbance in self-concept" is to assist the individual in identifying those activities or values that have formed the basis of the self-concept and to determine, with the client, alternative expressions of such important ego supports. In the past, and among the present very old, men have customarily had difficulty with their social adjustment to retirement. This was especially so for those who had no mate or spouse. Traditionally, it was the wife who established and maintained social ties. In contemporary society, however, all this has changed. Indeed, what the repercussions of an increasingly female work force will be and how they will cope with retirement when it is a commonplace event for them is a question still to be answered.

CONCLUSION

In this chapter, I have addressed major concepts that underlie emotional distress and disturbance in late life. Stressors, issues of self-esteem and self-concept erosion, and phase of life problems must all be considered as they impinge on satisfaction of human needs. Particular problems are often encountered related to bereavement, relocation to an institution, and retirement. Most often disturbances in sense of security, belonging, and self-esteem will accompany changes, transitions, and loss. Caregivers, therefore, should pay special attention to transitional stages in the individual's life passage. Such times provide an opportunity either for personal growth or deterioration. Caregivers can assist the individual to cope effectively and gain a sense of mastery.

3

Quality of Life Issues and Mental Health

Quality of life issues are those elements of daily life that provide satisfaction and comfort and support psychosocial needs. This chapter focuses on providing an institutional environment that is responsive to personal development and cultivation of interests and optimistic attitudes in staff and patients.

ENVIRONMENT

According to Funk and Wagnall (1983), environment is commonly assumed to be one's surroundings: the external circumstances, conditions, and things that affect the existence and development of an individual, organism, or group.

Therapeutic environments by definition must have healing properties that are curative, facilitate development, and enhance existence. In that sense, the terms *therapeutic* and *health* are synonymous. However, in the interest of making surroundings for our institutionalized elders more tolerable, even when not particularly therapeutic, I will discuss environment as it relates to mental health.

Given the diversity of needs and goals to which therapeutic environments are oriented, it is difficult to consider them collectively. However, it is probably safe to assume that the anticipated length of time in a setting is the most significant variable in relation to environmental impact. Another, less specific, consideration is the consistency of micro, and macroenvironmental control. In regard to issues of identity and autonomy, such consistency is particularly important. Where consistency is lacking, problems will occur. For example, when individuals are erratically given, or expected to take control of, elements in the environment beyond their capacity or interest, conflict—whether expressed or suppressed—is bound to arise. Certain features of an environment may also demand actions or responses beyond the capabilities of the individual. The more debilitated one becomes, the more environmental changes are likely to exceed capability. Environmental adaptations meant to facilitate self-care may be totally inappropriate for very impaired individuals. Even worse, failure is built into this situation by definition and, thus, continually erodes self-esteem. Within the microenvironment, for example, the most devastating, and perhaps frequent, struggle is seen with clothing: the individual cannot disrobe quickly enough to attend to his or her toileting needs. Incontinence, and the resulting shame and sense of defeat, are the consequences. Micro and macroenvironments, therefore, must be carefully designed to account for and counteract such consequences. They can make the difference in whether an individual is judged functionally competent or incompetent.

Personal Accoutrements as Environmental Barriers

An environment is euthenic when it is designed and controlled to improve human development. In this respect, should microenvironments be designed for and by the individual(s) who function within them for personal enhancement? Often aids to ambulation, hearing and visual deficits, even wheelchairs, result in distancing individuals from active participation and enjoyment of interaction. Ebersole and Hess (1990) provide in-depth studies of the effects of sensory deficits. It is sufficient here to remind caregivers that they may be significant.

Environmental Design for Elders   During renovation of a skilled nursing facility in Oregon, the innovative administrator decided to implement an architectural design that included "conversation coves" (Gamroth, 1983). These had been touted in the gerontologic literature as "angular alcoves that break up the sterile design of the long hall and invite 3 or 4 residents to stop and informally chat" (Cluff,

1975, p. 516). The Oregon facility decorated the alcoves with plants, wall hangings, and comfortable chairs. They were rarely used and it was never determined why they were not. This is only one example of well-intentioned actions that produced minimal benefits due to lack of input from the persons for which they were intended.

Protection for the Incompetent

Health professionals, sometimes out of democratic instincts, proclaim the value of nonsegregation of patients with dementia and socially disruptive behaviors. However, among patients there is a class system in which the most lucid form an aristocracy that implicitly and subtly discourages intrusion by the impaired. When living together on a daily basis, it is reasonable to expect that such a system would evolve. Social skills that enhance interpersonal relations are among the first to disappear in progressive dementias. It is not only personally threatening to see this happen to a peer but it is most difficult to be confronted with impolite, intrusive, and gross behaviors. From the perspective of the impaired individual, however, the macroenvironment itself may be perceived as threatening, confusing, and anxiety provoking, thus aggravating, rather than mediating, the impairment. Many facilities have developed special units for their psychologic and physical protection.

Adaptive Environments

Environmental responsiveness to the needs of patients has been a primary concern in some facilities. In Yakima, Washington, the Chalet Nursing Home, a family-owned 200-bed nursing home is designed particularly for individuals with various types of dementia. The total facility was planned with their safety in mind. While few facilities court these particularly difficult patients, it is refreshing to find some that do. Some of their special adaptations included:

A large grounds with high chain link fence surrounding it, to allow patients to wander at will.
A locked kitchen to prevent patients from entering and injuring themselves.
A large recreation room that included activities such as painting, puzzles with large pieces; card games; and select musical instruments such as harmonicas, drums, and a chord organ.
A garden where individuals could plant and harvest if they wished.
Fruit trees that were for patients' enjoyment.

A dog and a cat.
Small, comfortable benches placed strategically throughout the
building and the grounds.
Safety glass in mirrors and windows.
Safety electrical plugs.
Water heater thermostats lowered to tolerable water temperature.

While some residents were unable to take advantage of the opportunities provided for activity and gardening, it was surprising to find
many who retained some capacity for previous life activities and were
able to accomplish more than would ordinarily be expected given
their cognitive limitations. It is possible that, for residents, the lack of
structured expectations or demands and the comparative freedom
they experienced reduced anxiety sufficiently to maximize whatever
remaining skills they had.

There were undoubtedly other, less apparent modifications that
had been made to ensure the safety of residents while obviating the
need for restraints and allowing them full freedom of the facility.
Obviously, less time was needed for individual patient supervision. In
addition, markedly fewer medications were needed. Staff and patients
benefited greatly from the setting. Today, it provides a model of what
can be done wtih careful planning.

A segregated Alzheimer's nursing home was operationalized in
Morton Grove, Illinois. Hellen (1986) discusses some of the approaches used:

> We focus on companionship and supervision in a safe and therapeutic environ-
> ment. We have specific training for the staff to deal with Alzheimer's behavior
> (anxiety, non-verbal language, reversal of day/night schedule, etc.). That train-
> ing is for anyone who comes in contact with the patient, not just the nursing
> staff, but the housekeeping, maintenance and dietary staffs as well. We plan
> activities for seven days a week. Nurses' aides take over when the activity staff is
> not there. Another important consideration is weight and nutrition monitoring.
> Noneating can be a serious problem.
>
> We encourage patients to do as much as possible for themselves, to retain as
> normal a life as they can in a stress-free environment. We adapt to their needs
> rather than trying to press them into our environment. (Hellen, 1986, pp. 5–6)

A similar facility has been recently operationalized in Albuquerque,
New Mexico. Here, they have put lightweight screens over nonedible
plants to prevent patients from mistakenly picking and eating them.
Apparently, this minor adaptation is successful in deterring individuals from doing so.

While these adaptive facilities may not be as esthetically pleasing as
the usual nursing homes, it is also true that many facilities plan their

appearance to appeal to families who may be placing a parent. Of course, this is a legitimate concern and must be considered. Perhaps more effort must be made to educate families to evaluate facilities by other than carpets, chandeliers, and fine paintings on walls, however. The activity level of residents in a facility and the interactions of staff to staff, patient to staff, and patient to patient say more about a facility's philosophy and potential for quality of life than any of the external trappings, no matter how appealing or tasteful they are.

In regard to patients who require special care (e.g., patients who suffer from Alzheimer's disease or dementia), many institutions have developed care units specifically for them. However, in such a care unit, this caution must prevail: the unit must be designed for the special needs of the patients rather than simply as a means of separating them from the other patients who may be more lucid and easier to manage.

Schafer (1985) provides suggestions below for modifying the environment to make it more negotiable for cognitively impaired persons.

SIMPLIFIED ENVIRONMENTS

Reduce noise and distractions.

Provide environmental cues (clocks, calendars, photos of self, and color cues).

Eliminate prints on walls, floors, and furniture (they may be confusing or distracting).

Camouflage doorways with screens or room dividers (patients will seldom look behind them).

Place latch hooks one foot above eye level (patients will not look up to find them).

Decrease volume of TV.

Provide quiet places, headsets for music.

Use consistent names for rooms (lounge, TV, recreation, and dining room).

Use familiar terms (e.g., toilet, not WC or "john").

Privacy

In our affluent society, privacy and the size of individual space are indices of status. Individuals have become conditioned to expect that personal time and space will be respected. Yet there is extreme individual variability in the degree of privacy one finds necessary or desirable. Some behaviors common to collective living situations must be examined in relation to privacy needs. Is it possible that the "seclusion rooms" of the old state institutions were psychologically necessary as an escape into privacy, even if it was a privacy voyeuristically breached by the viewing window? Is a behavior, by definition, designed to provide distance between self and others? Is the result of certain behaviors isolation of the perpetrator? Does the behavior subside when the individual is separated from others? By such questions, I do not mean to suggest that aberrant or difficult behaviors are consciously designed for certain results. However, I do believe that when individuals live in an abnormal environment abnormal behaviors will be expressed to meet needs.

Roommates

Residents' influence on each other may make a significant impact on individual patient adaptation and overall effects of milieu. Seldom is sufficient consideration given to the roommate selection process. An individual living outside of an institution would not consider living with someone he or she hadn't selected. However, we do, and quite blithely, expect our elders, who may be even more entrenched in particular styles of living, to acclimate without resistance.

It may be that common problems roommates often express, such as decisions about heat or cold, windows open or closed, using the other's things or rummaging through them, playing the radio or TV at all hours, and constant prattling, are only superficial evidences of deeper feelings of intrusiveness, lack of privacy, and individual consideration. None of these issues are so different from those anyone may experience with significant others. When we are allowed little personal space or time to ourselves, we may complain about minor issues rather than facing larger ones. Even given careful consideration, the problems of having a roommate may emerge. It is probably wise to establish certain rules of conduct for roommates before problems arise and to exercise great care in roommate selection. Studies by Retsinas and Garrity (1985) and Wells and McDonald (1986) have shown that individuals in nursing homes tend to develop close relationships with persons of similar age, living in close proximity but not in the same room, and who have similar capacities and reciprocal needs. Factors to consider in selection of roommates include:

Introduction of individuals of similar age and capacities.
Discussion with each individual prior to assignment.
Discussion of specific life style issues significant to each.

Identifying mutual aid they may provide for each other.
Identifying times when each will have privacy.
Identifying individual staff that will be available to assist in problem
solving when differences arise.

Wells and McDonald (1986) found that among nursing home
residents one third expressed feelings of closeness to another resident
and two thirds said they had formed new friendships since entering
the facility. Of most interest is Wells and McDonald's finding that the
opportunity to provide mutual aid was significant in the development
of deep friendships. Apparently, the opportunity for friendships to
develop and flourish exists in many settings. The need to be needed is
consequential and should be respected.

Environmental Enhancement

Environmental cues have been discussed frequently enough and are
inexpensive enough to ensure general recognition and acceptance. Yet,
situations still exist where clocks, calendars, location of important
events, facility maps, and individual room identification are not in
evidence. This is purely neglect and requires only a concerted effort to
make immediate change.

While fully recognizing the difficulty in modifying ingrained methods of care, I would encourage staff to consider some of the suggestions offered and work toward implementing them.

While considering ways to implement suggestions and the difficulties that will be encountered in doing so, it is useful to remember
Wolanin and Phillips' (1981) recognition that the factors predictive
of and prodromal to confusion in the aged include disruption of usual
ADLs and distortion of time and space cues. Therefore, in those
situations where confusion can be prevented, the staff and the patient
will be gratified.

In addition, suggestions have been made to make the institutional
environment more communitylike. In pursuit of this ideal, Morganette (1987) suggested nature hikes for nursing home residents to
increase sensory awareness and interest in environment and to decrease separation from the natural world. For some persons, com-
munion with nature is essential to their sense of psychic renewal.
Unfortunately, little attention has been given to these needs; needs
that are not blatantly evident.

There are individuals who have not been outside an institution in
many years. Caregivers may assuage their conscience by believing
these individuals, if taken out, would become anxious and insecure.

But have the caregivers tried? Or is it too difficult for caregivers to provide these individuals the opportunity of being outside again?

Park rangers can often be enlisted to assist in a nature hike and be asked to provide experiences for the elders to hear, touch, smell, see, and taste. When individuals must be confined inside an institution, nature can be brought to them in the form of actual plants, leaves, pinecones, rocks, and other natural objects. If this seems too difficult, a first step may be to provide vibrant, colorful pictures of flowers, gardens, forests, oceans, and other natural beauties. Some of the Sierra Club calendars are lovely and would serve two purposes by keeping the elder in touch with the date and the beauties of nature.

Another unlikely, and somewhat controversial, means of individualizing the environment is to provide plush animals for residents. The critical issue in doing so is to view it as a comfort rather than as a childish condescension. Francis and Baly (1986), found that if they were self-selected and made available, but not recommended, the results were positive. Additional discussion of this study is found on pp. 68–69. Residents who chose plush animals often became quite attached to them, even naming them and commenting on how they enjoyed them. It was also observed that having a plush animal promoted interpersonal interaction, provided comfort, and improved interest in social activities. While all these elements are useful, it is well to remember Wolanin's comment: "In the absence of a comforting human interaction a plush animal may provide some small measure of comfort" (personal communication, 1985).

Almost all facilities have a library of some sort that is hardly ever noticed. Yet reading and discussion groups have been implemented in some settings successfully. Caregivers might find residents more interested in reading if there was a monthly trip to the community library for those who are able and desired reading materials brought to those who are unable to go to the library. Readings of great books and poetry might become a focus for discussion of philosophy and other interests that have lain dormant too long. Bond and Miller (1987) instituted regular reading groups and the building of a library in a long-term care facility. As a consequence of their intervention, they found residents interested and more interactive.

Psychosocial Needs and Mental Health

Quality of life issues in long-term care are significant in planning. A comprehensive review of recent studies related to the management of patients' psychosocial needs in institutional settings produced a large number of reported issues and strategies. It is important for nurses to remember that many of these are based on empirical data, anecdotal reports, or may be attempts to articulate grounded theory. Each setting and each group of patients will necessarily introduce different variables. To the extent possible, I would hope for replication of some of these findings or modified use to meet the needs experienced in a particular setting.

Hope   Hope as a life-sustaining force in the lives of the elderly has been given minimal attention. Farran (1987) found that in relatively healthy elders living in senior housing centers there was a statistically significant relationship between high levels of hope and social supports, interpersonal control, and religiosity. These data may be significant as guideposts for those caregivers dealing with elders who convey a sense of hopelessness.

Touch   Touch is an element often lacking in the lives of the elderly. Yet the "laying on of hands" has long been recognized for its healing and soothing effects. Kreiger's (1975) work has been used extensively in nursing and has shown the physiologic as well as psychologic benefits of touch. Often, we automatically reach out to someone who is anxious or in pain and may even find it difficult not to do so.

Caring touch has been used systematically in a nursing home setting as a cost-effective means to improve communication and quality of life of residents. Staff were trained to use caring touch frequently to become sensitive to the interaction between professional and client. The training model that prepared staff to use *caring touch* was based on Gendlin's focusing technique (in Sakauye & McDonald, 1987). The results not only showed significant increases in patient satisfaction but also had positive impact on staff morale.

Choice   Bueber and Hoffman (1987) studied elder residents and their satisfaction with nursing homes. As they hypothesized, those residents who perceived choices in the activities of daily living expressed greater satisfaction with their environment. They also found that the longer a resident stayed in a nursing home the less choice he or she perceived. Implications of this study are germane to quality of care and the well-being of residents in long-term care settings.

Resident Councils   Resident councils have been effective in focusing individuals both on staff and among patients to the specific desires of residents. Often, the first few meetings are simple gripe sessions, but this is necessary to clear the air for more productive efforts. Short meetings at least weekly are more likely to produce positive results than monthly meetings, however. Having a topic of focus each week and someone on staff to present and guide the discussion, can enhance facility management. For example, focus one session on diet, including: food preferences, meal schedules, recipe sharing, possibilities for resident assistance in meal preparation, and the possibility of an ethnic foods day. Occupational therapy is another topic for resident council discussion, especially in regard to products that allow residents to use their latent skills.

Many of these suggestions have been implemented in facilities I have visited, often in a highly refined manner. Typically, the noninvolved, depressed, or demented residents are least inclined to be represented. As a result, it might be useful to have separate resident council meetings. More functional residents thus will be able to make use of the full extent of their participation skills while least functional residents may have different levels of participation in which they are able to feel useful.

Usefulness   Ekerdt (1986) identified the work ethic and the need to keep busy as influential in the morale of the present generation of aged. Although much has been written about retirement transitional adjustments, little has been written purely on the need to keep busy as a moral expectation. Recently, I observed an old man whittling while on an airplane trip across country; almost a lost art! My grandmother always had something in her hands to knit, patch, mend, or crochet. If not that, the elders were making music with combs, bathtub bass, waterglasses, harmonicas, pianos, and fiddles. Even when hands were idle, bodies were rocking. One wonders if those were means for discharging what we call "nervous energy" in healthier ways than we presently use. In any case, it was rare to see anyone sit without "doing." If, indeed, the elders were a generation of doers, then we can easily apply that to them now.

In order to extrapolate to institutional settings, an individual's present level of "free energy" must be assessed. I am using this term to identify energy the individual has in excess of that needed to cope with the activities of daily living and any physical disabilities. If the individual is apathetic and inert after basic ADLs are completed, and displays fatigue, it is doubtful he or she has "free energy." If the individual is agitated or moving about, then it would be safe to speculate he or she has some energy that could be put to better use. In that case, Ekerdt's (1986) suggestions may be employed. These suggestions include the following:

BUSY ETHIC

Provide ways to keep busy in useful activity for those who feel morally compelled to do so. Encourage: assisting other clients who are disabled or confused; repairing items that are damaged or broken; and tutoring children in reading.

Provide productive leisure activities such as: quilt making, knitting, crocheting, gardening, tending plants or pets, decorating facility, planning celebrations (holidays, birthdays), and reciting poetry or singing.

Aasen (1987) states succinctly, "Opportunities to participate in activities consistent with personal talents, values and interests provide an opportunity for both decisional and behavioral control. Talents may be as varied as playing piano, gardening, or reading mail to others" (p. 23). To proceed in this effort, note the following suggestions:

- Identify issues in which resident has control, such as clothing, arrangement of personal items. Be aware that loss of some autonomy may be experienced as global loss and resident must be told areas in which he or she has decision-making power.
- Provide realistic opportunities for choice and alternative choices in areas of interest, such as which one of several books, newspapers, snacks, or music. Too many choices may have the negative effect of creating anxiety and a further loss of control.
- Build in opportunities to share personal talents, hobbies, and interests. Efforts must be made to identify these and residents should never be pressured to perform.
- Give information and rationale for situations in which resident has no control. (Aasen, 1987, pp. 25-27)

It would be a delight to see several items listed in every client's records that convey personal interests and talents as well as problems and disabilities.

Humor   Humor in healing and health care has been mentioned sporadically but with little consistent interest. Possibly the most familiar application of humor in healing is that reported by Cousins (1979) in *Anatomy of an Illness*. Quite recently, there have been many suggestions in the health care literature that attitudes and emotions have direct effects on immune response and healing. To date, however, there is no conclusive, irrefutable data that support this belief. Humor appeals to the absurd, is incongruous, ludicrous, and allows one to laugh at oneself without shattering one's ego. Some of the most humorous events occur in long-term care and the aged laugh with and at caregivers, as well as at themselves. Occasionally, I have found myself totally bewildered in a conversation because I have failed to recognize the wry humor of an aged communicant. Many of my favorite tales have as an underlying theme the very unpredictability and honesty of an aged person. For example, when Catherine said, "I *never* doubted my husband's faithfulness . . . but, I have heard that a man must have sex to be healthy . . . and he was *very* healthy." Or, when one old man in a nursing home was overheard telling another, "We agreed to stay together for the sake of the children, and now the little buggers have put us in the same home!" Because the aged have given so much joy and humor to those around them, perhaps caregivers can help them use it as a therapeutic tool to enhance life and hasten healing. It is important to remember, however, that humor may fall flat if an individual is in extreme discomfort or has some basic needs unmet.

Williams (1986) has written an excellent article on the therapeutic effects of humor in geriatric care. She notes very particular physiologic effects that enhance healing and energize:

Increased respirations.
Increased circulation.
Increased muscle tonus.
Production of endorphins.
Expansion and contraction of diaphragm.

Psychological effects of humor include:

Relaxation and stress reduction.
A temporary escape mechanism.
Interruption of the downward spiral of anxiety, tension, anger, or fear.
An acceptable expression of hostility.
Face saving.
A pleasant mind set.
Stimulation of insight.

Of course, there are certain times when humor is best used. Ascertaining those times is important as the ill use of humor can be destructive. Included below are aspects of the therapeutic application of humor.

THE THERAPEUTIC APPLICATION OF HUMOR

To assess conceptual ability of an individual.
To accept the expression of forbidden feelings.
To encourage spontaneity.
To interrupt negative cycles.
To activate physiologic response.
To reduce tension.
To create a sense of shared meanings or experience.
As a social lubricant.
To intervene in conflict.
To ease embarrassment.
As a social leveling mechanism.

Because the reaction to humor includes a complex psychophysical process, examples of its application may be useful.

Individuals who understand the incongruous relationship of manifest and latent meanings in puns are cognitively functioning on a rather high level. If they do not perceive the pun, they may be thinking only in concrete terms.

Ordinarily, individuals suppress the desire to laugh at the awkward behavior of someone who falls, but they can roar with laughter and not be censured when they watch slapstick comedy, which celebrates awkward and aggressive behavior. In this sense, humor is an acceptable outlet for some repressed aggressive feelings. In fact, when laughing, individuals can forget themselves and the image they may feel constrained to exhibit.

Negative cycles can become trenches, almost impossible to rise from. One lady, complaining about the abuses of her husband, was finally interrupted by the comment, "Weren't you tempted to hit him with a frying pan?" Such comments, however, must be used sparingly and only after the person has been allowed sufficient time to ventilate; otherwise, they can be perceived as cold and uncaring.

Laughter can be used for the deep breathing benefits or for any other of the physiologic effects that activate positive responses. The endogenously produced endorphins are natural substances with euphoric components. Caregivers are just learning some of the events that activate the production of these substances. Laughing seems to be one of them.

When tension rises, it is common to interrupt it with a laugh. An example of this is the joke about the man leaving the repair shop carrying a grandfather clock. As he rounds the corner, a lady bumps into him and shrieks, "Why don't you carry a watch like everyone else?"

Creating a sense of shared meaning is often a component of intimacy, frequently observed in lovers as they look at each other knowingly and laugh over some small event that does not seem humorous to anyone else. Much of this is related to a shared experience that brings them closer by the exclusion of others.

As a social lubricant, humor is often used by salespersons or speakers to "warm" the audience. It is meant to quickly establish rapport yet allows for the listener to retreat or advance without offense.

Intervention in conflict by the use of humor temporarily allows the participants to step back from their own invested position and see it more clearly. Two old ladies caught in an argument about seating in the dining room were distracted and began laughing as another quietly slid into the chair in dispute and began devouring the salad.

When embarrassed, humor may temporarily extricate an individual from the need to explain, and it may save face. The classic example of such action is attributed to Winston Churchill when a duchess exclaimed, "Sir Winston, you are drunk!" Reportedly, Churchill replied, "Yes, dear lady, but I'll be sober in the morning and you will still be ugly."

As a social leveling mechanism, humor is used to demonstrate that everyone of high or low status participates in certain ignominious situations. Scatalogic humor is often of this type.

Williams (1986) suggests several ways to stimulate humor in a long-term care setting:

Group sharing of funniest memories.
Masquerade parties.
Clowns.
Slapstick movies.
Reading joke books aloud.
Joke-telling sessions with prizes for those receiving the most applause.
April Fool's Day.

Eastern Onion simulations.
Read or tell amusing stories.

In conclusion, while humor must not be used indiscriminately, its therapeutic effects should not be neglected.

CREATIVE CARING

One of the greatest human needs is for self-expression of creative urges. Other related needs are for comfort and satisfaction. Modes of achieving expression of these urges vary widely at all ages. In late life, we would expect even more divergent and specialized interests to reflect a lifetime of choice and experience. In institutional settings, it is sometimes difficult to provide materials and space for certain self-expressive activities. Those suggested in the following pages have been tried successfully in various settings and may be adapted to the particular situations and constraints of a given setting.

Drama

Using drama to evoke new and perhaps more expressive modes of communication has been used in some long-term care settings. Dramatic improvisations can assist the elderly in different situations to express feelings engendered or to problem solve around issues they frequently encounter. Stern (1985) reported using drama in a workshop co-sponsored by Vista College in Berkeley, CA, and Hillhaven Convalescent in Oakland, CA. More information regarding this innovative approach to enhancing communication skills can be obtained by writing 2020 Milvia St., Berkeley, CA 94704.

Art

Working in groups, or individually if necessary, Rugh (1987) found expressive art an effective way for elders to express their inner experiences and feelings. The art activity seemed to provide an avenue for integration, personal revision of self-concept, and movement toward self-actualization. Rugh speculates that creative expression may be a more essential activity than has been generally thought in the lives of the elderly.

Ceiling Art   O'Connor (1987) has devised a method of enriching the environment of bed-bound patients by use of self-selected or

created art placed on the ceiling. She has dubbed this "ceiling therapy." Such creative efforts to enhance surroundings for immobilized
patients is encouraged.

Imagery

Imagery-based cognitive training techniques have been used successfully with elders. These techniques include visual imagery elaboration,
verbal judgment, and relaxation. Intuitive elders seem to benefit most
by this approach. Individuals are encouraged to visualize and describe
in detail situations in which they feel competent and relaxed.

Mythical Memories

Myths that provide solace and meaning are significant in the subjective world of demented persons. Gordon, Siegal, and Palmer (1987)
have used an oral history method to gather information that can
enhance the maintenance of self-concept and autonomy in the lives of
institutionalized, demented elders. Such persons retain some capacity
for happiness, tenderness, joy, and meaningful existence if the facility
provides the kind of care that accentuates these human qualities. By
encouraging patients to share their life story, with the admixture of
myth and reality they are able to retain a sense of their humanity and
uniqueness.

Music

Music has been recognized for its therapeutic effects since the time of
the ancient Greeks and Egyptians, yet caregivers have not given it the
credence needed to establish it as an essential therapeutic modality. In
this regard, an experience with a dying lady in an intensive care unit
early in my nursing career made a lasting impression. She entreated
the staff to get her Baroque music. She enjoyed this music and wanted
nothing more than to listen to it. The personal importance of her
dying request was not recognized or acted upon. We remained preoccupied with the trappings of our trade. She died, of course, without
the pleasure or solace the music would have given her.

Enough has been written about "canned music" and need not be
repeated here. However, careful selection of music in collaboration
with the client may have remarkable effects. Rhythms that are similar
to the heart beat generally have soothing effects. It is quite possible
that aggressive behaviors might be subdued by such music in an
environment that was quiet and nondemanding.

Glynn (1986) suggests some ways to use music effectively:

Music may stimulate physiologic response.
Music may enhance movement.
Emotions may be heightened and expression facilitated.
Group responses and bonding may be strengthened.
Self-esteem can be augmented when individuals sing or play an
    instrument.

Active participation can also be encouraged by asking individuals to
lead a song and to record performances.

Hydrotherapy

Activity and movement may be hampered in old age by arthritic
discomforts, parasthesias, and other disabilities. Indeed, Hallal
(1985) reports that the most frequently used nursing diagnosis is
"impaired physical mobility" and that it occurs to some extent in
79% of older patients. In a heated, buoyant pool such individuals can
be freed of their disabilities and discomforts. Though hydrotherapy
has been used extensively in rehabilitation services, pools are seldom
seen in long-term care settings. Cost and maintenance may be prohibitive. One facility adminstrator saw the potential value of a pool and
contracted with a nearby senior center, housed in the YMCA, for the
use of their pool one night a week. The benefits were reportedly well
worth the effort. Weinstein (1986) reports that aquatic activity has
the benefits of increasing social interaction, muscle strength and coordination, and comfort. All of these improvements were reflected in
improved ability to carry out the activities of daily living and thus
proved an overall benefit to the residents and the facility. One man
who had right hemiplegia had thoroughly rejected the offensive part
of his body that no longer obeyed him. After an hour in the pool he
said, "This is the first time I have felt whole."

Pets, Plants, and Plush Animals

Pet therapy has been approached from many directions and is usually
reported successful in increasing social interaction and life satisfaction.

A study by Bolin (1987) revealed the positive benefits of a companion pet and a strong support system in the process of grief resolution
following the death of a spouse. Neither one nor the other proved as
effective as both. This study did not test the introduction of a pet

during the grief process but only studied those persons who had bonded to a pet prior to the loss.

Pet therapy has been reported frequently in the literature. Recently, Connelly (1987) reported that even those persons suffering from the most advanced stages of Alzheimer's disease have responded positively to the presence of animals, especially dogs. He speculates that, as the gulf between patients and other persons widens, the patient can develop rapport with animals without fear of rejection or disinterest.

The reports of pet therapy have been impressive and have had many beneficial results but pets do require special care, adequate facilities, and consistent attention. Their inclusion in a facility can also prove dangerous to residents: for example, when a large dog bumps an individual whose gait is unstable. When, for whatever reasons, pets are not feasible within a setting, are dolls and plush animals acceptable substitutes?

Milton and Macphail (1985) reported that hospitalized elders expressed enjoyment of dolls and stuffed animals when they were made available to them. A staff nurse in a nursing home in Ogden, Utah reported that when dolls were brought into a facility, for patients who wanted them, some residents expressed disappointment because there were not enough dolls for everyone.

Francis and Baly (1986) reported on a facility that made a special event of bringing donated plush animals into a facility. A party was given and all the animals placed on a table for patient selection. Most of the patients chose a stuffed animal and gave it a name, often named after a pet they had in the past. They frequently carried their pets with them and put them on the bed while in their rooms. Those clients with limited mobility and reduced sensory capacities seemed most to appreciate having a plush animal companion. The results of this study showed the following benefits of plush animals in the facility:

Increased social interest.
Increased psychological well-being.
Increased mental functioning.
Increased life satisfaction.
Increased psychosocial functioning.
Decrease in depression.

While these results could not be considered precise, it was clear that the plush animals were generally beneficial. Similar results were also reported by Rodin and Langer (1977) when elders were given the care of self-selected plants. Caregivers might postulate that having something to care about that made no demands on elders and was unequivocally theirs were the significant factors in the success of these efforts.

A friend who was hospitalized told me a small stuffed dog was the most useful gift she received. When her neck or back ached, she could mold the stuffed animal and place it in just the right spot to relieve the pressure. The dog also provided something to talk about when she needed the relief of small talk with visitors. By trying not to treat institutionalized persons as infants, caregivers may have deprived them needlessly of comfort mechanisms.

Progressive Relaxation

Conceived by Edmond Jacobson in 1929, progressive relaxation is a method of teaching individuals to recognize tension by progressively tensing and relaxing various muscle groups throughout the entire body. Ultimately, with practice, the individual is able to consciously relax the entire body. When in a relaxed state, one may visualize positive changes, focus on strength and potential, and, most importantly, feel in control of reactions. Method instructions can be taped and used in small groups. Role modeling is also useful. Gillan (1983) reports success with reducing anxiety with a 75-year-old lady using progressive relaxation. The efficacy of this method has largely been ignored in work with the aged.

Progressive relaxation may be a useful behavioral approach to the management of the clinically significant problems of depression, anxiety, paranoia, and excessive pain.

Control of Anxiety and Pain with Progressive Relaxation   Pain and anxiety are sometimes considered together as they each amplify the other in the elderly. An important aspect of behavioral intervention in anxiety is the development of relaxation responses to be used in stressful situations. The first step is to identify clearly and in detail each situation that tends to create anxiety. There are myriad relaxation exercises for those who are anxious or experiencing pain. Their effectiveness will depend much on the cognitive focus the patient is able to sustain. Autogenic training packets are readily available and relatively easy to use (see Resources in appendices). As previously noted, many residents of long-term care have some degree of cognitive impairment and thus approaches must be modified and adapted creatively. There may need to be more visual representations of concepts, charts, and pleasant scenes to focus attention. Particular music that has been identified by residents as relaxing may be used adjunctively more frequently than usual. It is also important to discuss reasonable expectations rather than the complete alleviation of pain or anxiety. Rather than seeking a relaxed posture, some investigators have found physical activity useful. If this can be accomplished in rhythm with music, there may be an amplified benefit. Weldon and Yesavage (1982) documented the use of relaxation and other behavioral therapies in a group of patients with dementias of Alzheimer's type or of multiple infarct. These individuals were successfully able to learn muscle relaxation leading to self-hypnosis and trancelike states as well as practicing imagery. The group met for three one-hour sessions each week for three months. In addition to successfully mastering these techniques, the patients involved were significantly improved in activities of daily living. To induce sleep, one third of the patients were able to abandon the use of hypnotics and use relaxation techniques instead. This study has important implications for wider use of relaxation and other behavioral procedures in nursing homes.

THERAPEUTIC MODELS

As reported by Nick (1987), a *quality of life nursing care model* was developed at the College of Nursing, University of Illinois at Chicago and implemented in 3 nursing homes in Chicago. Decisional control and permanent assignment of nursing assistants to a specific group of residents were most frequently expressed as the most appreciated factors of the new model of care.

The therapeutic community model has also been tried successfully in some nursing homes and seems to bring about change. Community meetings daily, or at least twice weekly, in which patients and staff can discuss their needs and expectations within the setting form the core of a therapeutic community. Assuming responsibility for certain activities and unit functions is also an important aspect. Where this has been operationalized, residents with higher levels of function have become more assertive, expressive, and engaged in conflicts with other residents and staff. While these may increase ward problems in some circumstances, it is evidence of engagement in living as opposed to waiting to die. Staff selection would be critical to the success of such programs as the traditional lines of responsibility and authority must occasionally be modified or relinquished. Unfortunately, there are elements that preclude success that are common to nursing homes: high rates of staff turnover; staff and resident avoidance of areas of conflict; and staff and resident lack of authentic decision-making power, control, and self-direction.

In one small facility the young, female administrator was especially attentive to residents. She was frequently observed hugging a resident spontaneously. Awards and special recognition were also lavishly given. Residents were sought for counsel regarding problem situations and were carefully listened to. Children came to visit the facility in groups and with their parents and were warmly welcomed. Some children with profound disabilities were patients in the facility. Residents were encouraged to rock them and give them special attention. A poetry session I attended included persons with little talent and some who were quite talented. However, each person made his contribution and found satisfaction in it. The most unusual thing I observed was a large poster of a nude woman on the door of one man's room. It was obvious in many ways that this facility was designed to serve the interpersonal needs of the residents and that was the highest priority.

CONCLUSION

Quality of life for elders who are emotionally or mentally impaired has, by virtue of limited resources and imagination, often commanded little attention or priority in the delivery system of health care. Therefore, this chapter has focused on caregiver attitudes that contribute to life quality. Undoubtedly, such attitudes need to be cultivated and encouraged. Specific expressive activities for implementation also are addressed as are various aspects of environment that impinge on or are significant to life satisfaction, including suggested environmental enhancement strategies. While all these issues may seem an intolerable demand on already overburdened staff, when dealt with constructively, staff and patient enthusiasm and motivation are extended and positive benefits tend to increase exponentially.

4

Psychotherapeutic Strategies with the Elderly

Psychogeriatric care has many distinctions when compared to that of the general population receiving psychiatric care. Some models and considerations are discussed in this chapter in relation to the specific needs of the elderly client.

According to Dye (1985), the older adult brings to the treatment scene little awareness of stress as an agent of emotional disorder, sensory deficits that may alter communication potential, and little interest in or awareness of psychodynamic processes. Dye has identified the major issues of treatment as anomie, identity loss, mortality, and senescence. Most of the aged, however, are motivated to resolve problems, use their energies constructively, and find meaning in life. Successful treatment of the elderly has been accomplished through diverse approaches. However, traditional psychotherapeutic methods may exclude many elders due to cost and insufficient geropsychiatrists. As a result, geropsychiatric nurses and others with appropriate qualifications often manage much of the care.

THERAPEUTIC APPROACHES TO CARE OF THE AGED

There are many therapeutic strategies based upon sound psychologic theories that can be incorporated by nurses without intensive psychiatric training or extensive expertise in the care of the aged. This is fortunate as there are few highly trained professionals available to address the psychologic needs of long-term care residents. Seldom are there sufficient psychiatric consults recommended or solicited even in acute-care settings.

What are the therapeutic approaches to mental health problems of patients that can safely be used by staff with little training in psychology or psychiatry? Several suggestions will be provided with some cautions. Most important is identifying staff who are motivated to try new approaches and to learn about the emotional needs of the aged. The ideas instituted should have a universal appeal and be experienced by staff prior to implementation with patients. Below are listed psychotherapeutic intervention strategies.

PSYCHOTHERAPEUTIC INTERVENTION STRATEGIES

Individual psychotherapy.
Brief psychotherapy.
Crisis intervention.
Psychotropic drugs.
Group work.
Family groups.
Confidantes.
Peer counseling.
Reminiscing.
Life review.

The ability to listen thoughtfully and respond with empathy is essential and the first criterion of successful therapy. Some most enjoyable and successful communication exercises can accomplish this. One method is to have staff partners share their concerns with each other for a few minutes and gain feedback from the listening partner. Advice is discouraged and supportive comments encouraged. After each partner has experienced the importance of being fully engaged with a listening person, they are then instructed to share other significant events and feelings while the partner nonverbally demonstrates that he or she is not interested. The impact of this disinterest is usually felt strongly even though it is just an experiential exercise. The entire group then discusses their feelings and translates them into what patients may experience in such situations. Being a good listener is perhaps the most important skill a nurse can develop.

The ability to give meaningful feedback is another skill that can be practiced. Again, partners share some important hopes or concerns. The listening partner gives what he or she believes to be supportive and encouraging feedback to demonstrate attentiveness to what the other is saying. Monea (1978) devised a method for the sharing partner to respond, as well, to the listening partner's remarks. In this model, the sharing partner holds up a red card when feeling misunderstood and a green card when the listener has given useful or significant feedback.

When staff persons who are good listeners have been identified, there are other training programs designed to approach problems directly and in concrete terms. There are always at least two levels on which problems may be approached: the psychodynamic and the behavioral. In most cases, the behavioral approach will allow for referral for psychodynamic interventions when the resources are available and individual need is clearly apparent. Given the limited availability of well-prepared personnel, it is important to invent creative strategies for dealing with emotional issues.

There is great diversity of psychotherapeutic strategies that nurses can apply to care of the aged. Some broad guidelines that are generally applicable in the care of the aged include the following:

Be active and direct.
Recognize the variability of gerontic clients and adapt approach to the client's physical condition, previous level of function, and symptomatic history.
Be empathetic, not sympathetic.
Do not patronize.
Promote self-esteem through activities that enhance self-image.
Encourage involvement with others in community.
Accept the reality and validity of client's feelings.
Project an optimistic attitude.
Keep client mobile and involved with others.

Keeping these in mind when employing any specific therapeutic strategy will be useful.

Individual Psychotherapy

When individual psychotherapy is economically feasible and available to older persons and when therapists' attitudes are optimistic, results are positive. Unfortunately, there are only a select group of older persons who have had sufficient psychologic exposure to overcome their negative attitudes toward therapy, and have had sufficient economic resources and access to geropsychiatrists. Nurses with geropsychiatric expertise can also function effectively as therapists.

Brief Psychotherapy

Goldfarb and Turner (1953), as the first geropsychiatrists, and Brink (1976) have advocated brief (six weeks to three months) psychotherapy for elders. They recommend that transference issues be focused on the positive and that the therapist form a strong supportive alliance with the elder and set some practical short-term goals to be evaluated weekly.

Brief psychotherapy has been used effectively to achieve resolution of some emotional problems of the aged. Brink (1976) provides practical suggestions for such an approach:

Establish short-term goals that are measurable and visible, and that will give the client an immediate sense of progress and encouragement.

Cultivate warmth and positive feelings within the therapeutic alliance.

Share personal experiences, thoughts, and feelings with the client. Active involvement and sharing are useful.

Promote self-esteem of client through supportive comments, openness, and acceptance.

Develop your knowledge of client's total life context and life history. Provide practical supports.

An example from a student nurse at SFSU may suffice to highlight these suggestions.

A student was working with a very depressed old man. The family had given up trying to get him to do anything and were seriously considering placement in long-term care; he needed constant attention just to maintain his daily survival needs. The student encouraged the man to agree to see her weekly for several weeks. Her immediate goal was for visits only with no particular expectation of him. On the second visit, the student brought a picture of herself so the man could think about and plan his goals each week. The picture would serve to remind him of the upcoming visit. She encouraged him to discuss his first job and how the work world had changed since he was a young man. She gave him positive feedback on his persistence, ability to survive, and her growing enjoyment of the interviews with him. She made a special point of mentioning any specifics she learned from him. After several weeks, the depression began to lift. Throughout the course of the interviews, there was never any focus on the depression but only a focus on the potential of the individual.

Peer Counseling

Peer counseling is built on the expectation that many elders have developed considerable sensitivity to the issues of aging and are in the best position to provide support to other elders who may be less able to mobilize resources and express feelings. Sensitivity training is essential for peer counselors lest they project an image of superiority that further undermines the coping of the counsel recipient (Monea, 1978).

Nurses are often in the position of training peer counselors. Unfortunately, in most settings, peer counseling is an underdeveloped strategy. Obviously, it has much potential for resident peer counselors as well as for individuals receiving attention. Peer counseling is particularly effective with individuals suffering losses or adapting to institutionalization.

Crisis Intervention

Crisis intervention techniques can be used to deal with both large and small personal crises. The rules (summarized from Brink, 1976, p. 163) are simple and readily applicable.

1. Listen to the individual and encourage ventilation without unnecessary interruption.
2. Find out what about the crisis is troubling the individual the most seriously.
3. Provide some relief for the most troubling issues.
4. Recognize that crises activate old conflicts and issues that have been unresolved.
5. Note that crises intensify feelings of helplessness. Institute some ways for individual to gain control of some aspects of the crisis.
6. Identify previous coping mechanisms by identifying ways individual has handled similar situations in the past.
7. Leave the individual with information related to resources or supports. Write down phone numbers or names of persons that can provide immediate response if feelings become overwhelming. In institutional situations, identify an individual who is available to provide psychologic support.

The following is an example of how a crisis may be handled in an institutional setting.

Charles was hospitalized with pneumonia and was slightly disoriented due to oxygen deprivation, dehydration, and general debilitation. Though not totally alert, he was aware that his roommate died during the night. Charles had greatly feared his own death during this hospitalization. During the night, he thought he had heard his deceased wife calling him to join her. In the morning when the nurse entered his room, she found him extremely agitated and fearful. He vacillated between anger and tears. She sat with him, held his hand, and encouraged him to talk about his distress. He calmed slightly after ventilating and then said he could not possibly sleep again in that room. The nurse assured him that he would be transferred to another room. They discussed the choices he had regarding a new room and he chose one with a window overlooking the water. Then they discussed his fear of death. He was able to relate it to the painful manner in which his wife had died. The nurse brought in the results of his last sputum culture which demonstrated that he was recovering from the pneumococcal infection. Later the nurse assisted him in the room transfer and assured him that she would alert the night nurse to his previous difficult night and that he could call her if he felt the need or began to feel frightened again.

This example may present an ideal resolution rarely found in institutional settings. Nonetheless, with some thought and creative action, crisis situations can be at least partially resolved and the individual made more comfortable.

Psychotropic Drug Use

Psychotropic drug use will be dealt with in greater depth later in this chapter. I mention it here only to focus on this most used and abused of therapeutic interventions. Seldom is drug usage alone therapeutic. To be successful, it must be combined with a suitable, nonchemical curative strategy. In addition, nursing observations are critical to successful monitoring and management of psychotropic drug therapies.

Group Work with the Aged

Group work with the aged is a strategy that has been employed effectively by persons with little formal training. The therapeutic effectiveness of such efforts is dependent upon appropriate selection of patients in accordance with their needs, supervision of group leaders, and clear guidelines for particular types of groups. Coleaders are often used to enhance effectiveness. In addition, the input of other residents in the group often has profound effects in terms of providing understanding and encouragement. Who better than another resident can fully empathize with the situation? Suggestions for specific groups and guidelines can also be found later in this chapter.

Family Support Groups

Family support groups can be found in many communities and facilities. Even though "You and Your Aging Parent" may be a topic of interest and need, often it is difficult for them to get away from immediate responsibilities in order to attend. Some of the most effective community groups provide respite and transportation services. Support groups have two major elements: first, ventilation and feeling expression; second, mutual problem solving. Either component without the other is likely to be less effective.

For the families of elders in long-term care, support groups have been particularly successful in helping them work out feelings of guilt and failure (Richards, 1986). Chenitz (1979) found it was useful to have a group leader from outside the facility as families may fear reprisal focused on their loved one if they complain about quality of care. Also, it is helpful to include the elder in some family group meetings.

Confidantes/Confidants

Over two decades ago, Lowenthal and Haven (1968) identified the significance of a confidante in the maintenance of mental health. Since then, Berkman and Syme (1979) and others have corroborated the importance of an individual who can be counted on to provide nonjudgmental emotional sustenance. Not only is it comforting but the Berkman and Syme study demonstrated decreased morbidity and mortality among the sample who had identified a strong confidant.

Reminiscence

The inclination to reminisce has been used effectively for individuals or for groups of aged persons. The usability of this mode of interaction lies in the universality of the phenomenon and the ease with which even very disturbed or demented persons can find interest in sharing their memories or telling their stories. The greatest value lies in the fact that it is based on patients' remaining strengths rather than their deficits. In addition, it has the side benefits of increasing staff knowledge about the patient as well as increasing the individual's self-esteem. Specific psychotherapeutic applications of memories will be discussed later in the chapter.

This brief description of various psychotherapeutic strategies that have proved successful with the aged is meant to alert nurses to a range of strategies that they may employ.

PRINCIPLES OF PSYCHOGERIATRIC DRUG USAGE

Management of emotional problems and psychiatric disorders by use of medications has become a first-line strategy in care of the aged. Therefore, nurses must be well informed to monitor adequately. Even though only 12.4% of the population is over age 65, they consume 30% of all prescribed medications. Noninstitutionalized individuals over the age of 65 take an average of five to eight drugs daily; the most common being psychotropics, analgesics, and diuretics. Barely more than half the aged studied by Kiernan and Isaacs (1981) had accurate knowledge of their medications and none informed their physicians of over-the-counter preparations they were taking. On an average, aged persons are given 13 prescriptions per year and are seven times more likely to have an adverse reaction than younger adults. After age 80, the risk of adverse reactions triples. In addition, old persons are hospitalized for adverse drug reactions twice as often as those under age 60. Nurses must be acutely aware of medication effects and reactions.

As recorded by Ebersole and Hess (1985), Spencer et al. (1986), and Yanchick (1985), the physiologic changes of aging most usually cited that alter response to drugs include:

Absorption: Increased gastric pH
Decreased gastric motility
Decreased gastric fluid volume
Increased gastric emptying time
Decreased mesenteric blood flow
Decreased number of absorbing cells

In effect, changes in absorption response result in altered ionization; slowed as well as decreased absorption, dissolution and destruction of drugs; and increased destruction of acid labile drugs.

Distribution: Increased body fat
Reduced muscle mass
Decreased serum albumin
Decreased total body water

In effect, changes in distribution response result in altered lipid solubility; concentration of dispersion in various tissues and higher peak concentrations of drugs; prolonged half-life and excessive accumulation; and more free drug not bound to plasma proteins.

Metabolism: Altered liver function
              Decline in hepatic blood flow

In effect, changes in metabolism response result in a reduction in liver microsomal drug metabolizing activity. Due to the complexity of metabolic pathways and liver function, it is difficult to assess the efficacy of hepatic metabolism in the aged.

Excretion: Decreased glomerular filtration rate
              Decreased total renal plasma flow
              Altered tubular excretory capacity

In effect, changes in excretion response result in higher, more sustained blood levels of drugs; and excessive accumulation and toxicity.

Few physicians have actually had specific training in geriatric medicine. Beyond that, old persons are known to use over-the-counter preparations, borrow medications from each other, and use old medications that may have been prescribed for what they consider a similar problem. Some self-medicate with alcohol or preparations containing a high percentage of alcohol in addition to other substances they are consuming. Considering such factors, it is surprising there are not more adverse reactions reported (See Appendices for Gerontologic Pharmacologic Principles).

A disproportionate number of the drugs used by the elderly are psychotropics. Psychotropic medications are particularly hazardous for the aged individual whose ability to absorb, distribute, metabolize, and excrete drugs are compromised to some extent by the aging process. Many psychologic conditions for which these drugs are used may, in fact, be iatrogenically induced responses to other drugs and, further, may produce an idiosyncratic response due to incompatibility with other prescribed substances.

Yanchick (1985) has developed a table of drugs (Table 4.1) that are known to cause psychiatric symptoms when taken by older persons.

If caregivers are to more judiciously use drugs in the management of mental health problems of the aged, two major factors must be addressed:

1. A reevaluation of prescribing habits in which symptoms are often treated with drugs prior to knowledge of etiology.
2. A more sophisticated knowledge and understanding of the multiplicity of factors that can alter drug activity: certain disease states, genetics, concomitant drug use, sex, nutritional status,

TABLE 4.1	Drugs That Cause Psychiatric Symptoms

Drugs	Symptoms
Hypoglycemics Antihypertensives Phenothiazines Antidepressants Narcotic analgesics Antiarrhythmics	Nervousness, Apprehension, Irritability, Disorientation, Dizziness, Syncope
Cortisone Reserpine	Severe depression
Digitalis (toxic levels)	Arrhythmias, Agitation, Confusion, Disorientation, Dizziness, Apathy, Depression, Headache, Hallucinations
CNS depressants (major and minor tranquilizers, sedatives, hypnotics, alcohol, methyldopa, reserpine, antidepressants, narcotic analgesics	Lethargy, memory problems, perceptual disorders, delusions, agitation, panic, confusion
Anticholinergics (atropine, major tranquilizers, antidepressants, antiparkinsonian drugs)	Confusion, blurred vision, agitation, disorientation, impaired memory
Propranolol	Nightmares
Quinidine	Vertigo, tinnitus, headache
Procainamide	Manic behavior, giddiness, psychosis, hallucinations
Lithium toxicity	Blurred vision, slurred speech, ataxia, tremors

Adapted from Yanchick, 1985.
Source: From V. Yanchick. (1985). Drug therapy. In C. Dye (Ed.), *Assessment and Intervention in Geropsychiatric Nursing*. Orlando: Grune and Stratton.

biologic and biochemical changes, stress, environment, and bio-rhythms.

The sheer number of drugs and the complexity of human response to them requires specialized knowledge. (See Table 4.2 for Nursing Principles of Administering Psychotropic Drugs to the Aged.) Nurses

TABLE 4.2 Nursing Principles for Administering Psychotropic Drugs to the Aged

Nursing responsibilities

1. Accurate observation of need should guide decisions regarding drugs. Inexact impressions are dangerous.
2. Patient education and observation for potentially hazardous side effects are essential.
3. Minimum amounts of medication should be used and increased only when necessary.
4. Sufficient time should be given to assessing response to a drug rather than prematurely switching to another.
5. Conferences with physicians regarding specific reason for selecting and prescribing a certain drug facilitate appropriate drug usage.
6. Alert physicians to the total drug profile of an individual—including OTCs that are habitually used and alcohol intake. Hazardous interactions are frequent.
7. Encourage periodic lab tests to monitor cumulative toxicity.
8. Encourage physicians to discontinue all but life-sustaining medications for the first week of hospital admission. Medications may be the source of symptoms.
9. Use interpersonal contact and comfort measures before resorting to the use of hypnotics or minor tranquilizers.
10. Accurate recording of drugs given and reactions is important.

Source: From V. Yanchick. (1985). Drug therapy. In C. Dye (Ed.), *Assessment and Intervention in Geropsychiatric Nursing*. Orlando: Grune and Stratton.

must be prepared to understand the major categories of drugs and responses to them and to become very familiar with the commonly used drugs. Often, a careful review of the client's drug history and medical problems will reveal the source of present symptomatology. In addition, below are listed questions that should be considered prior to initiating psychotropic drug therapy:

- What are the medical conditions that may produce psychiatric symptoms?
- What are the current medications being taken or that have been taken within the last month?
- What nonprescription medications are usually taken or are presently being used routinely?
- What is the pattern and extent of social drug use:
  Alcohol?
  Cigarettes?
  Coffee?
  Other?

- What is the client's nutritional status?
- Are there significant alterations in function of:
  Liver?
  Kidney?
  Thyroid?
  Neurologic system?
- Are other drugs currently being taken that may adversely interact with the psychotropics under consideration? (Yanchick, 1985)

Whenever psychotropic drug therapy is initiated, it is important to follow the four guidelines listed below:

1. Complete alleviation of symptoms is an unrealistic goal; in most cases, a drug dosage that would abolish symptoms would produce harmful side effects.
2. Whenever possible, only one drug at a time should be added to a client's therapeutic regimen.
3. The beginning dose of most psychotropic drugs should be reduced by 30–50% for an elderly person. Dosage can then be titrated slowly to achieve the maximum benefit at the cost of least side effects.
4. *Periodic attempts should be made to further reduce the dosage or discontinue the medication entirely* (Yanchick, 1985).

DRUG MANAGEMENT OF
SELECTED NEUROEMOTIONAL PROBLEMS

Depression

Tricyclic antidepressants (such as imipramine and doxepin) are the most widely used drugs in the treatment of depression. It is postulated that they inhibit the uptake of such biogenic amines as dopamine, tryptamine, norepinephrine, and serotonin (neurotransmitters) thus increasing the availability of these mood altering substances. Due to variances in the effects of the drugs in this group, they should be selected carefully after determining the plasma levels of serotonin and norepinephrine and considering the sedative and anticholinergic effects. Drug selection and dosage titration are ordinarily not the responsibility of the nurse but patient education and the observation of reactions and responses are definitely a nursing responsibility. Suggestions for proper use and precautions include:

- Offering medications with food to decrease the possibility of gastric upset.
- Scheduling medications with ½ dose at the evening meal and the remainder at bedtime to maximize the benefits of the sedative effects.
- Educating the aged individual to expect that maximum benefits will likely take four to six weeks to occur.
- Drinking alcohol must be avoided while on antidepressants.
- Liquid medication must not be mixed with grape juice or carbonated beverages as effectiveness will be decreased.
- As hypotension is a frequent reaction, the client must be educated to rise slowly from lying to sitting and then to a standing position.

Frequent side effects include blurred vision, constipation, urinary retention, arrhythmias, delirium, tremors, dry mouth, nausea, and increased desire for sweets. Since many of these propensities commonly exist among the aged, careful observation is essential (Oppeneer & Vervoren, 1983).

Anxiety

The benzodiazepines (such as diazepam) are considered the preferred drugs for treatment of anxiety in older adults because they are less likely to interact adversely with the metabolism of other drugs. They can be used as sedative/hypnotics as well as antianxiety agents. The following cautions should be observed:

- Clients with depression, epilepsy, drug dependency, narrow angle glaucoma, and pulmonary, renal or hepatic disease must be evaluated with great care.
- Adverse interactions are likely to occur with alcohol, anesthetics, CNS depressants, MAO inhibitors, cimetidine or tricyclic antidepressants.
- Common side effects include light-headedness, drowsiness, fatigue, headache, ataxia, depression, blurred vision, skin rash, unusual excitement, nervousness or irritability (paradoxical reactions), bradycardia, and breathing difficulties.

Psychoses

Psychotic people grow old and psychoses can occur in older persons though functional psychoses without a physiologic base rarely occur for the first time in old age. However, there is a growing concern with the casual prescribing of antipsychotics for old persons.

Tardive Dyskinesia   Tardive dyskinesia is an irreversible syndrome that develops from long-term use of major tranquilizers. It is a disorder to which older persons seem generally more susceptible. It is noticeable by abnormal facial movements, such as cheek-puffing or pursing and smacking of the lips. Rhythmic and involuntary movements of the mouth and tongue make chewing and swallowing difficult. Other parts of the body may also be involved. Careful vigilance for the appearance of these symptoms and immediate withdrawal of the offending medication is critical. It occurs most commonly in females and persons with a history of brain damage. Quite obviously, then, persons with Alzheimer's disease or other organic dementias are at high risk of developing this problem if given antipsychotic medications. The potential dangers, complications, and side effects of these medications must be discussed with the client and family and used judiciously.

Neuroleptic Malignant Syndrome   The neuroleptic malignant syndrome is an uncommon but serious reaction characterized by an elevated temperature and extrapyramidal symptoms. Other symptoms of neuroleptic malignant syndrome include autonomic instability, confusion, incontinence, diphoresis, and agitation. Addonzio (1987) found that haloperidol was the most common neuroleptic identified in these cases. It is estimated that from 0.4 to 1.4% of aged patients on neuroleptics develop this syndrome which is fatal in 20 to 30% of cases. The medical complications of the disorder include cardiac problems, pneumonia, pulmonary emboli, and renal failure. The Addonzio study supports the need for caution in the prescription of neuroleptic drugs in treatment of the elderly.

Frequently, the phenothiazines (e.g., Thorazine®) and butyrophenones (Haldol®) will be the drug of choice for an older psychotic person, in spite of the admonitions listed below. Apparently, these drugs act by interfering with the transmission of impulses in the limbic and extrapyramidal systems. When administered to psychotic patients, the resultant action is to normalize mood, thought, and behavior. Admonitions regarding the use of these drugs include:

• Small doses with delayed increases—maximum drug effects may not be reached for several weeks.
• Discontinuation of the drug must be monitored by a physician for withdrawal reactions.

- Medication in liquid form should be taken with juice, milk, or carbonated beverages. Care must be taken to avoid getting the undiluted substance on the skin as a rash may occur.
- Hypotensive precautions should be taken.
- Medication effects will be negated if taken within an hour of taking antacids or antidiarrheals.
- Avoid overheating exercise, hot weather, and hot baths as the medication tends to induce hyperthermia.
- Warn patient that urine may turn a reddish-brown color.
- Photosensitivity will occur; therefore, protect client from bright sun.
- Drug incompatibilities need to be monitored carefully.
- Side effects include muscle spasms; restlessness; shuffling gait; ticlike movements of head, face, mouth, and neck; tremulousness; visual changes; skin rash; yellowing of eyes and skin; sore throat; hypotension; decreased perspiration; blurred vision; constipation; dry mouth; nasal congestion; difficult urination; decreased libido and sexual ability.

Insomnia

In old age, normal sleep changes can be distressing and when exacerbated by discomfort, worry, or illness the older person is likely to seek a soporific. Prior to instituting any chemical means of assistance, nurses must take a client's sleep history, determine sleep patterns, and any factors that have recently impinged on the individual's life style. Considerable effort should be exerted to avoid the use of medications. There are still many questions about their overall efficacy and safety. The disruption of normal sleep patterns and the tendency to produce oversedation, incontinence, paradoxical stimulation, hypotension, and dependency are serious deterrents. When sleep medications are necessary, the benzodiazepines and chloral hydrate are most effective. As the benzodiazapines were discussed in relation to anxiety, the precautions related to chloral hydrate are noted here.

- Capsules must be swallowed whole accompanied by a full glass of liquid to decrease gastric upset.
- Physical dependence can occur and rapid withdrawal of medication may be dangerous.
- Should be used with caution in the presence of cardiac, renal, hepatic, or gastric disorders.
- Monitor for compatibility with other drugs.
- Side effects include shortness of breath and irregular heartbeat

(symptoms of overdose); skin rash; hallucinations; paradoxical excitement; mental confusion; nausea and vomiting; stomach pain; clumsiness; lightheadedness; drowsiness; and a feeling of hangover. (Oppeneer & Vervoren, 1983)

It has been estimated that drug-induced changes in mental status account for as many as 16% of the cases of confusion or altered mentation that require hospitalization. Unfortunately, it is frequently overlooked as a cause. Drugs that commonly cause mental status changes in the elderly have been identified by Berlinger and Spector (1984) (refer to Table 4.1). Todd (1986) also reported on drugs that may, in fact, be the source of confusion and emotional distress. The drugs listed in Table 4.1 frequently create patient problems. Keeping a check list to determine the date and frequency of reactions ascribed to any of these drugs is helpful for the nurse to determine future drug interventions. The drug regimens of nursing home patients consume much of the time of professional nursing staff as they administer, record, and evaluate. Rovner (1987) has shown that two simple changes can reduce costs and release registered nurses (RNs) to other functions that may be vital and make better use of their professional skills. He recommends the following:

• Reduce the number of times per day a medication is given, considering its known pharmacokinetics.
• Reorganize the dose-interval schedules of the drugs comprising the total drug regimen.

Nurses, particularly those in nursing homes, have a great deal of responsibility regarding scheduling, administration, and observation of the effects of drugs. In many situations, an astute nurse is most critical to safe and appropriate drug therapy.

REMINISCENCE

The need to talk about and integrate life events occurs at all ages but, in old age, it takes on special meaning. Reminiscing allows one to develop a sense of continuity and meaning related to the whole life span. Some families, and caregivers, devalue reminiscing as an exercise in self-indulgence, ego stroking, or avoidance of immediate issues. In fact, it is vital to the maintenance of self-concept, core values, conflict resolution, and personal security (Ebersole, 1976; Ebersole, Burnside, & Monea, 1979; Ebersole & Hess, 1981). The usual psychiatric nursing diagnoses leading to the application of reminiscent strategies are: (1) potential disturbance in values/beliefs; (2) spiritual distress and despair (anomie, loss of meaning and purpose); and (3) disturbed identity processes related to individuation. Some ways to instigate therapeutic reminiscing are summarized in Tables 4.3 and 4.4.

Life Review

The concept of life review as a basic developmental process during adulthood, and particularly old age, was first introduced by Butler (1963) to explain a particular type of reminiscence he observed among old persons at St. Elizabeth's psychiatric hospital in Washington, D.C. From his perspective as a clinical psychiatrist, he observed how troubled old persons used repeated, often ruminative, verbalizations of their remote memories in an attempt to achieve understanding and a resolution of internalized conflicts. There was an obsessive quality to this action that often frustrated listeners and caused them to persuade, if possible, the elder to desist in order to pay more attention to the present and less to the past. Butler gave validity to the process and showed how it is really a manifestation congruent with psychoanalytic goals: ventilation, exploration, elaboration, catharsis, acceptance, and integration. Because it can be such a painful process and so closely resembles that of psychoanalysis, some nurses have been loath

TABLE 4.3   Specific Ways to Activate Memories

Recording life story for family or significant others.
Identifying personal legacy: products, contributions, talents, qualities.
Making scrapbooks.
Reviewing photo albums.
Identifying rituals of security and comfort.
Developing a work history.
Reviewing life's turning points, which can be mapped out as a road.
Initiating fantasy trips to follow an alternate road.
Resolving suppressed grief issues.
Identifying cohort with historic events.
Compiling life histories of significant persons.
Stimulating sensory/cognitive centers.
Stimulating memory chains.
Inventorying significant items, and determining their significance and disposition upon death.
Identifying favorite recipes, dietary history.
Entertainment.

Source: From P. Ebersole and P. Hess. (1985). *Toward Healthy Aging: Human Needs and Nursing Response*, 2nd Ed. St. Louis: C. V. Mosby.

TABLE 4.4   Guidelines for Dealing with Memories

Never disapprove but try to understand meaning of event.

Don't challenge accuracy of memories because all memories shift over time and are influenced by emotions.

Ask questions that do not require specific answers, e.g., "What year did you start school?" (no); "What do you remember about your first day at school?" (yes).

When you are getting bored with repetition, ask for detailed explanation of event, e.g., "You have told me about when your father bought the horse, tell me about you and the horse."

Try to focus on the person as the central character in any event described, e.g., "What were you doing then?", or "What did you think about that?", or "How did you feel at the time?"

Sometimes bring the person back to the present: How does he or she feel or think about that event now? What does it mean to him or her? How has it influenced his or her life?

When individual talks about a painful event, listen carefully, don't verbally reassure, and give time for long pauses without interrupting. Touch, hug, or hold the client if it feels right to you. Ask how he or she managed and who helped out?

Always work toward goal of increasing self-esteem of individual by recognizing his or her individuality. No one precisely like that person will ever exist again.

Share some of your own memories as long as it assists the client in becoming more expressive.

Source: From P. Ebersole and P. Hess. (1985). *Toward Healthy Aging: Human Needs and Nursing Response*, 2nd Ed. St. Louis: C. V. Mosby.

to deal with it. Nonetheless, nurses should follow the lead of the client. If they are in a state of readiness for life review, it is safe to encourage its expression. Guidelines for life-review therapy are listed in Table 4.5.

Life review is, in fact, vital to achieving a sense of self, core values, and security in a world of capricious and sometimes traumatic events. Indeed, the need to understand and search for meaning through introspection and validation is itself the source of personal and family myth.

Myth and Mid-Life Review.   Because life review of the elderly can seem an extraordinarily complex and difficult intervention, it is helpful to consider mid-life review as a precursor. In mid-life, one usually confronts a sense of mortality, as well as the dawning awareness that one does not get what one believes one deserves or has earned. As a result, there may come a sense of victimization or relief. Whichever holds true, it is profoundly moving to discover one's personal insignificance in the affairs of the world. The erosion of the "dream" of greatness that healthy youth held as a perpetual reality and motivation for striving is also confronted in mid-life. To a large extent, satisfaction in old age depends on how one reconstructs expectations and modi-

TABLE 4.5   Guidelines for Life-Review Therapy

Alert aged persons to the characteristics and normality of the life-review process.
Provide opportunities for aged persons to recapitulate events in their lives; e.g.,
  What has most influenced the course of your life?
  Who has most influenced the course of your life?
Assist aged persons to view their life experiences in a broader or different context;
  e.g.,
    As you explain your regrets, can you think of other factors that contributed to
      those events?
    How would you have changed your life then?
    What factors influenced your course of action?
    What would you do differently now?
Facilitate connections between past hopes, present events, and future expectations.
Be aware that the process may be carried out sporadically over several months. It is a
  painful examination of the past and is sometimes avoided.

fies the sense of self throughout the mid-life "crisis." Because this
"crisis" is recurrent, its intensity increases each time a major disjuncture in expectations occurs, or when values are questioned; thus, the
focus on mid-life as a critical time of review and revision of self-
concept toward healthy aging. In fact, while life review begins in youth
and continues throughout life for most persons, its urgency seems to
increase with age. Below are listed particularly relevant principles and
processes of life review.

PRINCIPLES AND PROCESS OF LIFE REVIEW

Readiness for life-review is a result of many factors and
should not be forced. When one is ready, its expression
should be encouraged.

Do not make interpretations and make every effort to
remain nonjudgmental either in a positive or negative
manner.

Encourage the client to express feelings and meanings related to events.

Recognize and encourage movement through the following
processes.

Ventilation is the initial, often ruminative, attempt to resolve an issue that is troubling the client. The issue is

often related to an erosion of self-concept and, as such, produces spiritual unrest and an erosion of self-esteem.

Exploration is the further discussion instituted by an interested and inquiring listener. This involves clarification and articulation of the event and moves beyond the repetitious, ruminative mode perpetuated by the internal troubled dialogue.

Elaboration requires more detailed description. Questions are meant to reproduce the essence of the experience in all its sensory impact, feelings, and impressions. At this stage, the challenge for the nurse is to keep the focus and avoid excessive circumstantiality.

Catharsis is the release of psychic energies through the expression of suppressed feelings that relate to the objectionable or disintegrative experience. At this stage, a nurse must be prepared to follow with the client into the "darker," more conflictive side of his or her nature, providing comfort by presence but not hindering the process by soothing comments.

Acceptance, in whole or part, will be achieved when catharsis has been sufficient.

Integration can be facilitated, hastened, and enhanced by the nurse who continues to explore the individual's values, beliefs, fantasies, dreams, and personal myths.

In general, the goal of life-review therapy is to release energy and create a sense of integrity related to one's life as lived. In this respect, Georgemiller and Maloney's (1984) efforts to use life-review in a therapeutic way as they worked with independent, highly functional elderly persons in senior centers is significant. Their methodology specifically involved interested members in a series of structured Life-Review Workshops (LRW). Each workshop series consisted of seven meetings of 90 minutes each. Each meeting provided some information related to various aspects of developing an autobiography. The second part of each meeting, however, was experiential and consisted of group sharing of autobiographical vignettes. Topics included developmental issues, religiosity, life purpose, stepping stones in life, significant people contributing to development of each, development of beliefs and values, significant life crises, attitudes toward death, and transcendental experiences. Control groups were devoted to activities and discussion of general issues of interest identified by the members.

The only significant difference that emerged between the groups was that the LRW groups became increasingly aware of their own mortality but without developing a more positive outlook about death. While this study may have been disappointing to the investigators who anticipated a more positive outcome, it does reinforce the assumption that genuine life review is self-initiated and can, at best, be supported and facilitated by others.

GROUP STRATEGIES WITH THE AGED

Group strategies with elders have been used both because of their effectiveness in patient outcomes and also because of their economical use of personnel and resources.

Maintaining a flexible group program that is responsive to the unique needs of older persons is a challenge in the management of a geriatric psychiatric inpatient unit. Clear definitions of the purpose of a group are essential so that patients may be placed into groups that best meet their needs. Patients need to be evaluated and selected for appropriate groups based upon capabilities, needs, moods, affective expression, thought processes, orientation, memory, impulse control, judgment, degree of insight, and motor activity. Groups that may be considered to meet various needs include: sensory, cognitive, and motor stimulation; reorientation; education and leisure counseling; problem solving skills; socialization and support; and grief counseling (Farran, 1987).

Keys to the success of these groups lie in patient assessment and selection, staff education in group conduct and process, and regularly scheduled supervision of group leaders. In regard to the establishment of group goals, there are five major foci.

1. Activity and mastery work groups that foster opportunities for reaching out, touching, exploration of materials, tension channeling, and ego mastery.
2. Cognitive and information groups that emphasize educational models, family life models, and occupational or recreational skills.
3. Interpersonal and socialization groups that focus on security, a sense of belonging, and companionship.
4. Relationship and experiential groups that work toward social habilitation.
5. Uncovering and introspective groups that emphasize personality growth.

Burnside (1984) has compiled a particularly useful source of information on numerous types of groups with the aged. Nurses who desire to further investigate group types for the aged, should refer to this book.

Yalom's Principles

Yalom (1970) created a classic text on the use of group therapy. He identified 12 curative components of therapeutic groups that one may expect as natural developments in the course of a group. The specific components are:

- Altruism: the development of concern for the good of others in the group without thought of reward for the action.
- Group cohesiveness: the ability of the group to work toward mutual goals and support each other, sometimes in opposition to leaders.
- Universality: the development of group awareness that many feelings and experiences in life are common to all members.
- Interpersonal learning: input from others in the group that share their knowledge.
- Interpersonal learning: output to others in the group that conveys knowledge of the speaker.
- Guidance: mutual problem solving and identification of a range of options for a given situation.
- Catharsis: sharing feelings that have been bound in alienation and nonacceptability.
- Identification: cohort or group accomplishments that bring pride to members.
- Family reenactment: attribution of family member characteristics to group leaders or members; corrective input is essential.
- Insight: awareness of self and motivations that have previously been elusive.
- Instillation of hope: meanings and goals derived from the group experience that provide growth perspectives.
- Existential factors: focus on present moments of shared joys and sorrows, which includes the ability to relinquish some past and future concerns.

If staff can be trained and oriented to these curative components of groups, it will provide a method of guiding and evaluating.

Due to limitation of resources and lack of available psychogeriatric professionals, group activities and therapies have been the predominant mode of meeting psychosocial needs of elderly institutionalized patients. Though many reports are anecdotal and nonreplicated, it seems that groups do provide positive benefits to what might otherwise remain a drab and alienated existence. Given the belief that groups are helpful to promoting socialization, self-esteem, some life satisfaction, and often increased functional capacity, I will review classic group strategies that have seemed to produce positive results.

Reminiscence, Reality Orientation, and Remotivation Groups

The "three Rs of therapeutics" remain the most frequently applied therapeutic group modalities. There are as many variations as there are individuals using them. Many empirical studies have been done but little solid research exists to reinforce any particular approach as best. It is most important to remember that aged persons are likely to respond positively to any attempts to touch their lives in a caring and empathetic manner.

Reminiscence Groups   Life-review, as explained earlier, is the most intense form of reminiscence activity and has the most therapeutic potential for personal growth, but there are many other forms of reminiscence that are therapeutic in other ways. It is probably one of the most versatile and most natural methods of working with the elderly in groups for some of the following reasons:

1. The natural tendency to talk about one's life experiences can be quite readily facilitated by even an inexperienced group leader.
2. There are enough commonly experienced life events to facilitate a sense of connection and mutual engagement when exploring these.
3. Reviewing life events is a means of focusing attention, exercising the mind, and stimulating memories that have lain dormant. Reminiscence thus creates memory chains and may increase cognitive capacity.
4. Even the very demented individual has some memory of earlier times and these can be used to stimulate a sense of self and recapture some self-esteem.
5. The discussion of early life events allows the listener to better understand the era and epoch of experience from which the elder gained his or her identity.
6. Groups of aged persons can develop a sense of solidarity and continuity based on their common participation in certain historically significant events.

There are many ways the tendency to reminisce can be used as a tool of group therapy, socialization, remotivation, assessment, and reality orientation. It is versatile because it is ubiquitous, natural, and embodies the whole of one's conscious life experience. Table 4.4 on p. 90 identifies relevant guidelines and suggestions.

Reality Orientation Groups   Reality orientation (RO) was conceptually formulated and initiated in the Tuscaloosa, Alabama Veteran's Administration Hospital in 1965 as a structured method of orienting confused elderly on an ongoing basis (Taulbee & Folsom, 1966). Its goals were to motivate staff toward therapeutic involvement with confused elderly and to improve memory and orientation of clients with cognitive impairment. Prior to that time, no serious attention had been paid to improving RO by enhancing memory. It soon became apparent that such efforts proved beneficial to participating clients and staff.

   In the years that followed, RO had many proponents and detractors. Those who found it effective, modified and elaborated their methodology and developed specific types and levels of RO. Encourage students to use any method available to orient older confused persons to environmental parameters and expectations that are vital to survival and function. In general, RO is most useful for persons with psychiatric nursing diagnoses that include perceptual/cognitive impairment in intelligence, memory, attention, and orientation. Currently, RO remains an intervention widely used with confused elderly. Certain specific interventions that have proved useful over time are listed below. See Table 4.6 for RO guidelines.

PRINCIPLES OF REALITY ORIENTATION

- Provide a supportive, accepting relationship; feelings are more easily discerned than thoughts.
- Recognize and verbally validate any contributions offered. There must be room for dignity in failures as well as successes.
- Reality orientation must be consistently applied by all personnel and relevant to issues of daily coping.
- The environment must provide orienting cues, such as clocks, calendars, names on doors, pictorial symbols, and other means of providing information.
- Multiple sensory approaches are useful to enhance learning and response. Avoid overload of input, however.
- Reminiscing about early life events may be easier than the present and increases patient's self-esteem.
- Staff involvement must be ongoing. Where it has been discontinued, patients soon regress.

TABLE 4.6 Differences Between Remotivation, Resocialization, and Reality Orientation

Reality orientation	Resocialization	Remotivation
1. Correct position or relation with the existing situation in a community. Maximum use of assets.	1. Continuation of reality living situation in a community	1. Orientation to reality for community living; present oriented
2. Called reality orientation and classroom reality orientation program	2. Called discussion group or resocialization to differentiate between a social function instead of a therapeutic need	2. Called remotivation
3. Structured	3. Unstructured	3. Definite structure
4. Refreshments and/or food may be served for identification	4. Refreshments served	4. Refreshments not served
5. Appreciation of the work of the world. Constantly reminded of who he is, where he is, why he is here, and what is expected of him	5. Appreciation of the work of the world. Reliving happy experiences. Encourages participation in home activities relating to subject	5. Appreciation of the work of the group stimulates the desire to return to function in society
6. Class range from 3 to 5, depending on degree/level of confusion or disorientation from any cause	6. Group range from 5 to 17, depending on mental and physical capabilities	6. Group size: 5 to 12
7. Meeting ½ hour daily at same time in same place	7. Meetings three times weekly for ½ to 1 hour	7. Meeting once to twice weekly for an hour
8. Planned procedure: reality-centered objects	8. No planned topic; group centered feelings	8. Preselected and reality-centered objects
9. Response of resident is responsibility of teacher	9. Clarification and interpretation is responsibility of leader	9. No exploration of feelings
10. Periodic reality orientation test pertaining to residents' level of confusion or disorientation	10. Periodic progress notes pertaining to residents' enjoyment and improvements	10. Progress ratings

(continued)

TABLE 4.6 (continued)

Reality orientation	Resocialization	Remotivation
11. Emphasis on time, place, person orientation	11. Any topic freely discussed	11. Topic: no discussion of religion, politics, or death
12. Use of portion of mind function still intact	12. Vast stockpile of memories and experiences	12. Untouched area of the mind
13. Resident greeted by name, thanked for coming, and extend hand shake and/or physical contact according to attitude approach in group	13. Resident greeted on arrival, thanked, and extended a handshake upon leaving	13. No physical contact permitted. Acceptance and acknowledgment of everyone's contribution
14. Conducted by trained aides and activity assistants	14. Conducted by RN, LPN/LVN, aides, and program assistants	14. Conducted by trained psychiatric aides

Source: Adapted by permission of The Gerontologist/the Journal of Gerontology, from E. Barns, A. Sack, and H. Shore, The Gerontologist 13(1973):513.

Remotivation Remotivation is a method of rekindling interest in the world, activating one's potential for participation, and combating the effects of institutionalization. It was initially conceptualized by Smith (1952) in an effort to apply learning theory to the rehabilitation of chronically ill and institutionalized mental patients (Long, 1962). Later, when it was seen as a particular mode of intervening with the institutionalized elderly, its goal was modified to enhance interest and quality of life rather than to return to production within the community. The appeal of remotivation therapy was immediate and clear: it could be done in groups and with the relatively untrained personnel common to institutional settings. The structured expectation and guidelines for remotivation (see Table 4.6) ensured that the issues addressed would be manageable. With elders, however, they are usually applied in a much more eclectic manner and with considerable warmth and caring demonstrated by the group leaders.

Because remotivation deals with specific individuals with unique problems, I encourage nurses to devise their own methods or techniques, and to remain sensitive to the moment. One particularly stimulating method is to focus on nature and natural phenomena that elders do not encounter in an institutional setting. For example, a student brought a collection of sea shells for discussion. The stimulation of multiple senses as the elder looks, listens, holds, and smells the objects may have deep impact. Listening to the sea shell stirs dormant memories of doing so as a child and the wonder he or she experienced. The symmetry and beauty of the shell reminds the elder of all the beauty and order inherent in nature. Other items that are especially meaningful include recordings of birds or other natural sounds, plants, spices, and colorful prints of interesting places. Something as common as a coffee grinder and coffee beans will stimulate a lively discussion.

When used with the elderly, remotivation therapy is for enhancing their interest and involvement in the world about them, whatever the setting may be. It is also useful as a second level of intervention with patients after they have advanced through basic RO. Butler and Lewis (1982) provide guidelines for instituting remotivation groups.

PRINCIPLES OF REMOTIVATION

Establish a warm and friendly relationship among group members.

Provide a bridge to reality through reading current events, sharing impressions of objects, focusing on the world of nature, and coping with the present situation.

Avoid emotionally laden issues. Working through those is not the purpose of these groups.

For specific structure of remotivation groups see Table 4.6.

Remotivation is most useful for persons who are apathetic, disinterested, and lacking stimulation. Psychiatric nursing diagnoses would include: emotional impairment, inappropriate levels of responsiveness, and self-care deficits.

CONCLUSION

This chapter has introduced the range of therapeutic strategies that are appropriate for the aged. In reality, all therapies useful for adults are suitable for the aged though some may be more effective with the modifications and applications suggested. In long-term care institutions, the aged are likely to receive little direct therapy; thus, group therapies have been suggested to overcome that lack. Particular attention must be paid to adapting the sophistication of the particular therapy to the abilities of the aged and to the capacity of the provider. As mentioned earlier, in situations where the individual is deprived of individualized attention, any one of these therapies is likely to produce positive results in terms of adaptation and life satisfaction.

5

Management of Common
Behavioral Problems

The management of behavioral problems in any setting in which the disturbed aged are encountered is a major consideration. In families, failure to manage such problems may result in institutionalization. In acute-care settings, when the client is often in a crisis state and receiving many treatments and medications, quite uncharacteristic behaviors may emerge or personality traits may be exaggerated. In long-term care setings, behavioral problems may arise from the nature of the setting, from misguided attempts to meet basic human needs, and from the disturbed mentation that is a frequent concomitant of institutionalization. Because each individual will have unique ways of acting out frustrations, specific needs must be considered when planning care. As such, this chapter examines the impact of milieu, staffing, and possible reasons for difficult behavioral problems. In addition, specific problems will be addressed individually with suggestions from the literature for dealing with them. Emphasized throughout, is this aim: any particular behavior must be examined within context and need as well as life history and previous coping patterns of the client. The goal is to provide guidelines for managing difficult behaviors while maintaining the dignity and individuality of the client. The preponderance of material in this chapter is related to clients in the long-term care setting as disturbances affect quality of life for an extended period of time.

IDENTIFYING PROBLEM BEHAVIORS

Actions identified as problem behaviors may be traced to many sources, both direct and indirect. There are often multiple, and sometimes obscure, reasons for disturbing actions but rarely a simple cause and effect. The "whys" are always more difficult to discern than the "whats." In the following section, I will explore issues that must be considered in seeking a solution to problem behaviors.

Whose Problem Is It?

It has been long assumed in child psychiatry that children exhibiting problem behaviors were usually mirroring the pathology of the family and, because of dependency needs, had become the symptom bearer or scapegoat for the entire group. It is not too outrageous to apply these same concepts to institutionalized elders, especially in long-term care where a pseudo-family and a subtle, yet intricate, social status system exists. In this respect, Golander's (1987) contribution to the literature lies in her precise identification of the underlying motives and myriad actions taking place "under the guise of passivity" in an Israeli nursing home. Is this then a problem of the milieu, the institution, the staff, the community, or of distorted national and local social priorities? Are we expecting an individual to wear a shoe that is designed for the convenience of the shoe salesman? Humans are amazingly adaptable, even very old humans. We find them surviving and sometimes enjoying the most contorted and contrived situations.

Who Is Affected by the Problem?

In an effort to determine the unseen components of a problem, caregivers must first look at the individuals affected by it in order to understand the underlying forces. For example, wandering is a great problem for an institutional administrator whose reputation for safe and protective care may indeed be "walking out the door" (Fennelly, 1982, Secure Care Systems, Inc.). It is also a problem for staff who will be blamed for not being alert enough to interfere with the "escape." Family may be furious and sue the institution if any mishap occurs. While various management strategies are discussed later in the text, caregivers should ask themselves who they are serving by detaining the individual who wants to wander outside?

Milieu Risk Factors

When attempting to identify precipitants to problem behaviors or to predict the risk factors in a setting, there are several critical elements that must be assessed.

Is the staffing adequate on all shifts?
How stable is the staffing?
Are expectations of staff and residents consistent?
Does the administrator make decisions and follow through?
Is staff morale high?
Is there time and space for privacy and "centering" oneself?
Are sensory adaptations made in the environment?
Is the environment safe?

In other words, is this a place in which a client could pursue some activities that give his or her life meaning? If it is not, then the setting must be modified. Attempting to treat festering social wounds with individual Band-Aids will only allow client problems to fulminate.

Determining the Source of the Problem

Among patients, problem behaviors often arise from inappropriate assessment and care plans, professional disinterest, ageism, social policy inequities, restrictive environments, and unstable staff. Some of these are remittable and some require major changes in national policy. On a more personal basis, behavioral and emotional problems of aging often arise from:

Basic need deprivation.
Depersonalization/loss of self-esteem.
Need for attention and recognition.
Need to be needed.
Life history of marginal adaptation.
History of mental health disorders.
Impaired cognitive capacity.

When considering problem behaviors, it is important to distinguish carefully the nature of the problem. Who is experiencing the problem? Are staff distressed? Other patients? Family? If caregivers understand the needs of the person expressing frustration, they may understand something of the problem. Behaviors that disturb the equanimity of the institutional environment may, in fact, add elements more resembling life stresses experienced in the larger community or they may make the environment intolerable for others. In this respect, it would be useful to survey the residents of a facility to identify the behaviors that they find particularly difficult to tolerate. For instance, patient arguments may be productive in keeping individuals interested in expressing their opinions and be indicative of a more lifelike institutional community. On the other hand, patients who threaten others must find alternate ways to express their anger or frustration.

Facility problems are frequently reflected in resident behaviors. For instance, with each change in administration in one facility, residents would become anxious and express their concern in various ways. Some would attempt to test the strength of the new administration by disrupting routines. When staff morale fell as a result, patient dissatisfaction rose. Because each patient is concerned about alliances and attention to personal needs, large turnover in staffing can create profound unease. However, when elderly clients in acute- and long-term care exhibit behaviors disruptive to the environment, staff, other patients, or any combination of these, it will be necessary to modify those behaviors. When implementing modification, consider these points:

Patterns of the behavior and the precipitants.
Staff actions and reactions to the behavior.
Clients' cognitive ability and responsibility for the action.
Environmental confusion and distractions.

While there are no recipes for resolution of problems caused by objectionable behavior, the following suggestions may also be helpful as a beginning point:

Immediately take the client to a quiet, calm place.
Discuss the problem with the client and determine his or her understanding of the difficulty.
Observe the client over several days and note the precipitants and patterns of behavior; modify the client's exposure to the trigger events.
Meet with staff to discuss their feelings, reactions, and possible modifications of their responses to the patient.

Hussian (1986) identified several severe behavioral problems that are especially difficult to tolerate in a congregate setting and has provided rationale for deciding when and how to address such problems. The following questions may assist staff to decide whether any intervention is necessary or whether the problem can and should be tolerated (adapted from Hussian, 1986, pp. 125–137).

RATIONALE FOR ADDRESSING MANAGEMENT PROBLEMS

If the answers to these questions are "yes," then action is justified.

Is the problem directly or indirectly damaging to the lives, health, and safety of the patient or those in the vicinity?

Is this behavior likely to elicit punitive measures by other patients or staff?

Does the behavior disrupt the unit milieu sufficiently to interfere with therapeutic endeavors?

Will interruption of the behavior, or treatments used to quell the behavior, interfere with therapeutic benefits of being on the unit; e.g., medications, restraints, or seclusion that, in effect, isolate the individual from benefit of therapy?

Is the amount of staff time used in correcting the problem at the sacrifice of more proactive, therapeutic activities on the unit? In other words, is the time invested likely to pay a reasonable return in benefits to the patient or the milieu?

Does the behavior frighten visitors to the unit or interfere with constructive social interaction with these visitors?

Does the behavior result in loss of materials or supplies or damage to property that is necessary or costly?

Does the behavior lead to avoidance of the person at all times, not just when the undesirable behavior is occurring?

Does the behavior prevent discharge to a less restrictive setting?

Does the frequency and intensity of this behavior erode staff morale and interfere with job satisfaction?

Prior to deciding on any intervention it is important to keep a record of frequency, duration, and intensity of the offensive behavior. These measures then provide a clear indication of the severity of the problem and can be used as a standard by which the relative success of interventions can be measured against the degree to which the behavior is extinguished.

One of the irritants that staff frequently mention is the sexual exhibitionism, including overt masturbation, of some patients. The previous general suggestions, if implemented, might extinguish the behavior if the client was given appropriate suggestions regarding where and when to masturbate. One staff member commented she could always handle such behavior by commenting, "Put that away, it's the smallest one I've ever seen." This only demonstrates the many distortions and preconceptions caregivers have about sexuality and points up the need to deal with it more seriously and sensitively as a basic human need.

Severe behavioral problems that tend to cause discomfort in the observer occur at relatively high rates in the geriatric population with dementing disorders. Because they are particularly difficult to manage, they will create all manner of reactions in the observer from rage, shame, and disgust to fear. Some problem behaviors are evidence of organ dysfunction that may be manifest in disruptive behavior before any physical manifestations are present.

Reasons for Behavioral Problems

Hussian (1986) has advanced six reasons for severe behavioral problems occurring more frequently in later life.

- Mentally and physically based organic disorders are manifest in disruptive behavior.
- Diminished or absent social networks deprive the person of corrective feedback and social reinforcement necessary for adaptive responding.
- The individual may be in a situation where little reward or positive response is given for acceptable behaviors.
- Low expectations of others and acceptance of dependent behaviors may reinforce disruptive behaviors.
- Diminished sensory acuity may be responsible for what appears to be inappropriate behavior or poor judgment.
- Central nervous system disorders may be evident by poor judgment and impaired impulse control.

BEHAVIORAL MANAGEMENT

While there is little reliable data regarding interventions in problematic behavior, Bootzin and Shadish (1986) contend that, at this stage, considering the enormity of need, it would be better to err by including interventions that might later prove not generally applicable than to set too stringent criteria. The success of an innovative approach in any particular setting may be due to any of several spurious causes. In addition, interventions designed for a given facility or resident may not be applicable or effective in other settings or with other individuals.

Behavioral Approaches to Enhance Mental Health

Effective behavioral approaches to mental health include not only traditional behavior modification techniques but biofeedback, modeling, and cognitive restructuring as well. General goals are to:

Alleviate human suffering.
Enhance human potential.
Improve functioning.
Increase skill.
Cultivate independence.
Increase satisfaction.

These can best be achieved when client and staff reach mutual agreement on the methods to be employed.

Behavioral approaches focus on specific data, are problem oriented, and clearly delineate direction and expected outcome. The client is given greater control over the outcome and major responsibility for achieving agreed upon goals. In regard to elderly populations, behavioral approaches have been used effectively with two types of symptoms (Richards & Thorpe, 1978; Patterson & Jackson, 1980). The first type involves socially significant behaviors (e.g., incontinence, inability to feed self, and impairments in activities of daily living) and are usually seen as problems more by staff than residents. The second type are clinically significant behaviors (e.g., anxiety, depression, and paranoia) that produce emotional discomfort for residents. Top priority should be given to the second type of problem. With relief of emotional distress, socially significant behaviors may be enhanced concomitantly.

Behavioral Management of Patients in Long-Term Care

Discussion of behavioral management of the psychogeriatric patient focuses primarily on patients in long-term care situations, whether mental health facilities or nursing homes. Some discussion and studies can also be extrapolated for use in counseling families regarding home care of elder members and could provide the basis for development of a select group of management protocols. Many similar problems are found in acute-care settings. However, because patients in such settings are usually acutely ill, receiving multiple medications, treatments, and tests, these suggestions may not be as applicable there.

Of particular concern is management of patients with emotional problems residing in nursing homes. While these settings tend to have the fewest mental health professionals available, it is estimated that some 60% of residents should have a primary diagnosis of mental disorder. This is not done because of reimbursement constraints discussed in Chapter One.

Two areas of assessment most often attended to in the aged are the neuropsychologic and the functional. In regard to functional assessment, Lawton and Storandt (1984) have added important dimensions to this concept. Attributes of the "good life" are indicated by positively assessed qualities in four major sectors: behavioral competence, psychological well-being, perceived quality of life, and objective environment.

- Behavioral competence is judged as that considered normally necessary in adapting to the external world and includes physical health, functional ability, cognitive competence, time usage, and social interaction.
- Psychological well-being is the personal feeling of satisfaction, or happiness, one feels about self in relation to the external world. The core of psychological well-being is self-esteem.
- Quality of life is a subjectively judged quality in relation to particular limited areas of interaction with the external world that are of value to the individual. Those areas that commonly contribute to or detract from quality of life are family, friends, work, housing, neighborhood, income, and recreational pursuits.
- Objective environment is the consensually judged quality of all that lies outside the individual. These are all the domains that are independent of the individual's single-minded perception and are subject to a high degree of consensus. They include the natural or man-made environment, geographical factors, racial character, average health, government, economic forces, and institutionalized social influences that impinge on the person.

The relationships among the sectors of the "good life" are not necessarily of equal significance or predominance. One may enhance one sector and influence the overall sense of satisfaction experienced. Thus, the holistic perspective is conceptually relevant. The repercussions of action or intervention are never singular but, like a pebble thrown in a lake, will extend outward in all directions in a negative or positive manner.

Unfortunately, however, an institutional environment is hard put to mimic the "good life" and, by its very nature, mitigates against consensual validation of the adequacy of such an environment.

Kane et al. (1986) identified certain individuals who survive better in institutional settings than others. These individuals are characterized by their general cantankerousness or "cussedness." Kane calls this the "curmudgeon factor" and considers it a positive sign of adaptive strength and personal security. It is sometimes predictive of longer survival. Therefore, an environment objectively considered deficient of life quality possibilities can be subjectively better tolerated by some individuals than others.

Assessment of the individual with a behavioral problem must precede a plan of action. All nurses are well indoctrinated in this process but when on the "firing line" sometimes respond in an obvious cause and effect mode. For instance, when Maude tears Kleenex into small bits and tucks them in her dresser drawer, the overt response is to remove the Kleenex or, when she is incontinent at night, to put her in a diaper.

Deitrich (1986) has suggested a thorough manner of assessing problems before instituting action. This assessment of behavioral problems is presented below.

ASSESSMENT OF BEHAVIORAL PROBLEMS

Note changes in behavior
   Illness may present as behavioral change
      Note irritability
      Isolated incidents of incontinence
      Abrupt withdrawal from activities
      Episodes of confusion
   Subtle changes indicate medical or psychiatric problems
      Biorhythmic or homeostatic alterations
      Family or nurse most likely to notice these
         Mild confusion
         Malaise
         Declining appetite or activity
         Insomnia
Assessment needs
   Thorough physical examination
   Observation of patient at different times of day

Observation of patient in various situations
Communicate with patient about the problem
Communicate with family about the problem
Discuss problem with other professionals
Describe behaviors specifically and carefully
Identify differences in patterns of behavior
Learn relationship to past history and habits

Deitrich suggests refraining from pharmaceutical intervention until the problem is clearly identified and other methods of intervention have been tried. An example may suffice to illustrate the point.

Irene seemed disinterested in breakfast, usually her favorite meal of the day. She had been incontinent during the night and seemed unaware of it. She was lethargic and resisted getting up. She seemed slightly disoriented to time and place. The staff wondered if she had suffered a transient ischemic attack (TIA) during the night.

Her physician was called and ordered routine lab work only to discover that she had a urinary tract infection. Remember, older persons may have an infectious process fulminating without a significant increase in temperature.

In addition, geriatric nurse practitioners have noted that many elders developing urinary tract or respiratory tract infections first show signs of confusion and malaise.

Behavioral problems associated with dementia are particularly difficult to deal with as the patient is often unable to intelligibly discuss feelings and concerns. Accurate and thorough assessment then becomes extremely important though sometimes neglected. The unremitting course of dementias of the Alzheimer's type generally follow a slow and progressive course with symptoms of cognitive disturbance most noticeable and with other symptoms that are characteristic of the areas of the brain most infiltrated with senile plaques and neurofibrillary tangles. When uncharacteristic behaviors or symptoms occur they must be investigated as elders with dementias are subject to all of the other problems concomitant with aging. The correction of superimposed disorders will ensure the opportunity for maximum function at whatever stage of Senile Dementia of the Alzheimer's Type (SDAT) the individual may have reached.

Deitrich (1986) has again provided useful directives for assessing the behavioral problems that may emerge in the demented patient. The DEMENTIA acronym in Table 5.1 will provide a useful guide to ensure that thorough assessment has been completed.

TABLE 5.1   Dementia Acronym

D	Drugs
	Psychotropics
	Polypharmacy
E	Emotional distress
	Depression
	Stress
	Bereavement
M	Metabolic/endocrine disorders
	Diabetes
	Hypothyroidism
	Dehydration
E	Environment/eyes/ears
	Changes in living situation
	Sensory losses
N	Nutritional
	Anemia, B12, Folic acid
	Alcoholism
	Constipation
	Anorexia
	Poor dentition
	Self-starvation
	Inability to purchase food
	Depression
T	Tumors
	Trauma
I	Infections
	Pneumonia
	Urinary tract
A	Acute illness
	Congestive Heart Failure
	Myocardial infarct
	Pulmonary Emboli

Deitrich, 1986; Coordinator, Gerontological Nurse
Practitioner Program, UCSF

Behavioral Modification as a Strategy

Behavior modification has been suggested as a successful approach in
the management of agitation, combativeness, multiple complaints,
multiple demands, yelling, abusive and threatening verbalizations,
self-stimulation, noncompliance, wandering, inappropriate voiding,
and inappropriate sexual behavior (Hussian, 1986). Considering that
many elders may have been deprived of consistent, caring, and corrective feedback for one reason or another, it may be useful to attempt
humanistically designed behavior modification strategies to extinguish

objectionable behaviors. Indeed, many behavioral problems persist because of a lack of such designs, including:

- The absence of positive consequences following appropriate behavior.
- The absence of discriminative stimuli to elicit appropriate behavior.
- The presence of aversive consequences following appropriate behavior.
- The presence of positive consequences following inappropriate or dependent behavior.
- The presence of inhibitory discriminative stimuli.

These contingencies and environmental events, many of them built into institutional function, shape geriatric responses and may lead to excessive, deficient, or "out-of-context" behaviors. An example may serve to demonstrate the point.

Olaf often stuffed towels and other objects into the toilet which, of course, caused the toilet to overflow and nurses and maintenance men to come running. The episodes provided some excitement and action in what might otherwise have been a dreary and boring existence. Olaf was strong, physically healthy, and capable of grooming himself and carrying out the activities of daily living with minimal assistance but his judgment was severely impaired by dementia of the Alzheimer's type. Olaf had once been a musician and had played a theater organ in the days of the silent movies but efforts of the activity therapist to interest him in music seemed to capture no attention. Usually, Olaf simply wandered around the facility and was hardly noticed. Episodes of stopping up the plumbing were rare and occurred only in his own bathroom. During January, the behavior seemed to increase and the staff held a conference regarding it. Most staff knew little about him except for his background as a musician. They did recognize that his excellent physical condition probably demanded some exercise. An exercise program was planned for him and he was given praise for completing it each day. He was also noted to be a loner and was included in a reminiscing group each week with the intent of providing some positive interactions with other patients. During the course of one of the groups, Olaf shared that his mother was often upset because he didn't pick up after himself when he was a child. An alert staff recognized the significance of that information and recalled that Olaf's mother had died at age 90 only three years before in January and that she had been his only known relative. It became easier then to understand Olaf's actions even though the reasons had never risen to his consciousness. He had always tried to please his mother. In mourning his mother and trying to please her, he would remember to pick things up but would throw them in the most convenient container, which happened to be the toilet bowl. A large orange hamper was put in his room and the staff trained him to put soiled towels and clothing in it. Because Olaf was the only one with an orange hamper, he felt special and faithfully used it. The undesirable behavior was extinguished and Olaf's quality of life was improved by some astute detective work on the part of the staff.

With the exception of extinguishing the undesired behavior, this example demonstrates several principles of behavior therapy. Olaf was no longer rewarded for inappropriate behavior but, instead, was given attention and experienced positive consequences of the more desirable behavior. In fact, Olaf demonstrated an idiosyncratic reaction to a specific psychic need. There are many more common problems for which caregivers have some guidelines to assist in understanding the problem and effecting resolution.

COMMON PATIENT MANAGEMENT PROBLEMS

There are no clear cut behavioral problems without numerous underlying factors and ways behavior is affected by others in the environment. Despite that caution, the problems that are particularly disruptive in a setting are usually addressed as if they were discrete entities. For example, the reader will recognize some methods that may be useful in a specific situation if adapted to the individual elder and the setting. In addition, many of the studies discussed have been conducted in long-term care settings where particularly difficult behaviors may become entrenched over time and deplete the quality of the environment for those living and working there.

The Alcoholic Elder

The National Institute on Alcohol Abuse and Alcoholism (NIAAA) believes that it is important to view alcohol problems of the elderly from a realistic perspective but, as yet, no one really knows the extent of alcoholism and related problems among the elderly. In fact, there is a distinct tendency toward underreporting of alcohol use among the elderly. Some reasons for this include:

Unawareness that drinking has become a problem.
Symptoms may not be associated with drinking.
Physicians and families are unable or unwilling to recognize the problem of elderly alcohol abuse.

To better understand this problem, Maddox, Robbins, and Rosenberg (1986) compiled the proceedings of an NIAAA conference at

Washington University in 1984. A profile of elderly alcoholics emerged that suggested they tend to be relatively free of other psychiatric disorders with the exception of cognitive impairment. Anecdotal evidence also showed that persons who rarely drank earlier in life sometimes relax prohibitions regarding alcohol consumption and may even develop abuse and dependency syndromes for the first time in late life. Women who have difficulty adjusting to the retirement of their husbands and the absence of children from the household are thought to be at particularly high risk of late onset alcohol problems. Only 1.4% of the elderly, compared with 3.9% of persons under 60 years of age, had been reported (DIS/DSM III) with a diagnosis of alcohol abuse or dependency.

An important consideration with the elderly alcoholic is the likelihood of medication interactions and incompatibilities that is much more a threat than among younger persons who imbibe excessively. In addition, many of the chronic, degenerative diseases of the aged may be exacerbated by the use of alcohol in excess.

In a majority of cases, late life alcoholics report psychosocial stressors precedent to problems with alcohol. Of 216 medical histories of elderly alcoholics reviewed by Finlayson, Hurt, Davis, and Morse (1987) many were found to have coexistent psychiatric problems. In particular, prescription drug abuse, organic brain syndrome (26%), atypical organic brain syndrome (19%), affective disorder (13%), and personality disorders (42%) were apparent. In light of these findings, the authors recommend careful psychiatric assessment of elderly alcoholics and exercise of restraint in the tendency to quickly relegate them to the diagnosis of alcoholism. In order to instigate effective treatment, correct diagnosis of the primary disorder is imperative.

The alcoholic elder is particularly amenable to treatment if the pattern behind the excess drinking is identified. Often, it is a response to social isolation, grief, pain and discomfort, insomnia, and depression. Typical Alcoholics Anonymous (AA) programs are useful methods of treatment. Strengthening the social network and reducing isolation is usually quite effective, as well. Providing satisfactory outlets for talents and instilling a feeling of being valued are extremely important. Some elders have sought treatment or been persuaded to accept treatment in intensive alcohol abuse programs on an inpatient basis. These report a greater success rate with elders than with younger clients. The outcome for treatment and recovery is optimistic, particularly for those who are late-life alcoholics and have developed that as a coping strategy to deal with the various problems encountered in the aging process.

Anxiety

Anxiety often arises from feelings of insecurity, powerlessness, and unpredictability. The elderly often complain of feeling nervous, upset, or uneasy. They may not identify the source of these feelings but they are demonstrated in restlessness, inattention, and confusion. At times, the anxiety may assume expression through compulsive channeling that may relieve the generalized, pervasive sense of impending doom. In those cases, it is temporarily more manageable but the real issue may be ignored. Below is a case study that illustrates this point.

Mrs. B. managed to handle her anxiety by focusing her attention on the time. She frequently got up at night and came to the nursing station to ask the correct time. She also kept an alarm clock under her pillow which she would reset to wake her every two hours. The staff were initially sympathetic with her need for attention but soon became annoyed with her and alternatively ignored or scolded her. Staff constantly reminded her that she was disturbing other patients on the unit, and did nothing to help her alter her behavior. It soon became apparent that Mrs. B. could not discontinue her irritating actions regarding the time and that it was an expression of some greater need. The nurse whom Mrs. B. most often sought out began to spend one half hour each day with her after breakfast in an attempt to establish a deeper relationship and discover the cause of the anxiety. After getting to know more of Mrs. B.'s history, the nurse learned that Mrs. B.'s husband had died in his sleep and Mrs. B. found him already cold beside her when she woke in the morning. The event had been so traumatic she had been unable to sleep for more than a few moments at a time for weeks after his death. When she was able to sleep again she began having nightmares about death. Her fear of dying in the same way had become an obsession. When the staff understood her death anxiety and her peculiar adaptation to cope with the stress, they developed a plan to help her deal with her grief and fear of dying. First, she was reassured that staff make nightly rounds each hour and that they would gently wake her if she wished. It was also decided that the nurse–patient relationship that had been established would be continued but the focus would shift to grief support. Active efforts would be made to encourage the expression of Mrs. B.'s feelings. Mrs. B. was gradually able to relinquish the alarm clock and requested that she not be wakened during the night. The relationship with the nurse allowed her to externalize feelings that had immobilized her and she was able to be discharged to her home. She continued to attend day care at the facility where her loneliness was assuaged. For further discussion of grief management see the section on bereavement in Chapter Two.

Aggression

Aggression is any act that causes or intends to cause damage or hurt to a person, animal, or object. Assaultive actions that are aggressive include striking, shoving, yanking, grabbing, pinching, kicking, biting, and throwing things.

Possibly, one of the most immediate causes of aggression in institutional settings is the lack of privacy, clearly defined personal territory, and personal space. Hospitalization tends to alter a person's territorial awareness. The need for one's own space becomes greater as the possibilities are diminished.

Behaviors that indicate subversive protection of thwarted territorial needs and thus indicate potential for violence if abruptly intruded upon include:

Withdrawal and retreat into self.
Pushing away from others.
Decreased eye contact.
Spreading things out around self.
Consistently sitting in the same place.
Arranging solid boundaries around the self.
Facing away from others in the room.
Increased sleeping.
Retreating into drugs.
Retreating into fantasies.
Withdrawal into reverie of previous times and places.
Exacerbation of habits, activities, or manners that disgust others.

Gordon (1985) has constructed an extensive list of behaviors that indicate potential for violence. The defining characteristics include the following:

Clenched fists, angry expressions, rigid posture.
Hostile verbalizations.
Boasting about abuse in the past.
Marked increase in motor activity.
Destruction of objects in the environment.
Possession of destructive items.
Expressions of rage.
Self-destructive behavior.
Substance abuse.
Suspicion of others' motives.
Fulminating anxiety.
Fear of self and others.
Inability to verbalize or recognize feelings.
High situational stress.
Manic excitement.
Provocative acts.

Those persons with some diminished cognitive capacities and judgment may have the most difficult time controlling angry feelings. Yet, many theorists believe that personality bents as reflected in life history are more predictive of potential violence than any present impingement on personal space.

Threatened aggression and altercations among institutionalized psychogeriatric patients disrupts the environment and intensifies anxiety and agitation among residents and staff. Donat (1986) surveyed reports of incidents regarding altercations among residents of an institution and has provided useful facts and suggestions as listed below.

ALTERCATIONS AMONG INSTITUTIONALIZED PSYCHOGERIATRIC PATIENTS

Facts:

9–12% of fractures are result of intentional actions by other residents.

Younger, stronger patients more assaultive: equally true of male or female.

Assaulted patients are described as intrusive, cognitively impaired, meddlesome, wanderers, ambulatory, and invading personal space.

61% of altercations occur between 3–8 p.m. (cortisol levels?)

Sites included:
dayroom 45%
hallways 25%
bathrooms 11%
dining room 8%
bedrooms 6%
other 6%

Suggestions:

Increase staffing in places and times where altercations occur most frequently.

Assign victims and aggressors to different day rooms.

Supervise dayrooms.

Increase structured activities during critical hours.

Provide behavioral training for the cognitively impaired.

Teach self-control to aggressors.

Provide other ways to express frustration and anger.

Aggression as Communication   O'Connor (1985) has given particular attention to aggressive threats and assaultive actions as attempts to communicate. In attempting to understand the message, it is useful to separate aggression into types:

- *Benign aggression* is in self-defense or protection of vital interests. It may be seen as life-sustaining as it is a response to threat.
- *Malignant aggression* is destructiveness and cruelty for no other purpose and is seen only in humans.
- *Pseudo-aggression* is playful or accidental harm that was not intended.

O'Connor (1985, pp. 2–3) provides a case study to illustrate the relationship between communication and aggression.

> Mr. T. is a 68-year-old obese male, post CVA with hemiparesis, severe COPD, and diverticula of the throat. He has frequent coughing and choking episodes. Considered medically fragile, he has resided on the long-term care unit of a veterans hospital for several years.
> Mr. T. has poor impulse control and frequently, when the unit is busy or there is a shortage of staff, becomes demanding. He sometimes refuses to get out of bed, occasionally defecates in bed or spills his urinal on the bed or the floor. He often avoids eye contact, but sometimes will look directly at you when speaking.
> He has daily physical therapy and looks forward to it as it gives him some sense of control and mastery, i.e., he walks in the parallel bars, has specific goals to work toward, and also the hope that he will improve enough to be discharged to a senior handicapped apartment.
> One morning, his usual nursing assistant had the day off. Mr. T. was struggling with various items in his bedside drawer to find his glasses. The nurse walked in and said, "It's time to get ready." She rummaged through his drawers and threw out several candy bars, saying, "No wonder you never lose weight." She found his glasses and gave them to him.
> Then she gave him a basin of water and insisted he wash himself. She left, calling, "I'll be back in a few minutes." He was partially successful. The nurse returned much later, saying, "Oh, Charlie, you're not done yet? I'll finish it." He throws the washcloth on the floor because he can't reach his armpit. As the nurse finishes, Mr. T. states he wants to be on time for physical therapy. The nurse says "Uh-huh." As she bent over to place his foot in his pajamas, he kicked her in the breast.

When considering the apparent provocations of this incident, it will be helpful to use Boettcher's (1983) *Assaultive Incident Assessment Tool.* The components must each be assessed individually (see Table 5.2). By incorporating these needs, caregivers might readily alter the previous case study to prevent the assaultive incident, see below.

TABLE 5.2 Assaultive Incident Assessment Tool

Need	Deterrant to Meeting Need
Territory	Invasion of physical, psychologic space
Communication	Lack of interpersonal attention, interest, or listening
Self-esteem	Lack of respect or being shamed, humiliated, and insulted
Safety/security	Absence of concern for safety or protection from harm
Autonomy	Deprived of decision making or control
Self-pacing	Urged beyond one's capacity, rushed or hurried
Personal identity	Personal items disregarded
Comfort	Inattention to discomfort that is present or inflicted
Knowledge	Confusing information or none related to expectations

Adapted from Boettcher, 1983

Mr. T. is approached by the relief nurse. She introduces herself and asks how he is feeling. She explains that she would like to assist him in preparing for physical therapy and inquires about his progress in therapy. Noticing that he is rummaging in his drawer, she asks if she can assist him. If he agreed, she would carefully help him look for his glasses. When she discovered the candy bars, there would be no need to comment or touch them. If dietary restrictions are imperative, she would set aside a later time to talk to him about foods that are important and help him decide what substitutes would be acceptable. In giving him the basin of water, she would ask what temperature he preferred, ask him to do what he could in washing, and give him a specific time when she would return to help him finish.

Such obvious changes in approach are simple to accomplish. However, because of inattention or lack of staff motivation, they may not be carried out. In addition, when staff are overloaded and frustrated, even the most obvious care improvements may seem impractical. To overcome such obstacles to improving care, staff will need education and attention to their needs. Regular staff meetings to vent frustrations in a safe and supportive environment will also reduce staff need to scapegoat patients.

One large and energetic 70-year-old man with a history of destructive behaviors and aggressive actions was admitted to a veterans hospital. His very presence was frightening to patients and the knowledge of his history kept staff at a distance. In general, he was alienated and abandoned. In order to attract some attention, he began making loud threats and demands. In one case, he made a gesture of hitting an orderly without actually doing so. From a distant perspective, it is easy to see his need for communication and attention. However, if he is frightening people in the environment, such recognition may be more difficult. A geriatric clinical specialist met with staff and discussed her perception of his actions to enhance their empathy for him. She also met with the patient daily and contracted with him each day not to hurt anyone. She set up an exercise program for him to productively use some of his energy. Her personal attention to his needs and encouragement of verbal expression of his many reasons for anger helped him control overt expression of his rage (O'Connor, 1985).

Hussian (1986) presents combativeness as an expression of agitation that may arise from four sources:

Frequently observed as one of the first signs of Alzheimer's disease or a related disorder.
Startle response and reflexive striking out secondary to distortions, misperceptions, or hallucinatory processes.
A method of gaining attention or preferential treatment in an institution.
As a symptom of physical illness, particularly congestive heart failure, mild myocardial infarct, or marked abnormalities in glucose metabolism.

Catastrophic Reactions   *Catastrophic reactions* may initiate violence with no identifiable precipitants. They are triggered by environmental demands or frustrations in excess of the individual's capacity to cope. Demented persons are particularly subject to such reactions.

Even though a lack of impulse control may be a notable symptom of dementias and hypoxia, it is possible to diminish the tendency to strike out by reducing demands and environmental stimulation. For example, "time out" is a respected, and often effective, method of behavioral conditioning. A major reason may be the temporary relief of expectations that are producing frustration. "Time out" may also be part of a contractual agreement with the patient. In this respect, the nurse may tell the patient, "When you are having trouble controlling yourself, we will take you to your room and stay with you there until you feel able to control yourself." In its most extreme form, restraints can be considered "time out" for the patient who is then temporarily relieved of the burden of self-control.

Cuizon-Saiz (1988) reports a nursing intervention of similar content below.

Mr. O. frequently threatened staff during episodes of anger and agitation. This usually occurred when staff were giving personal care. The nursing assistants consistently dealt with this by saying, "Mr. O., when you are ready I shall come back." This was often repeated several times before Mr. O. calmed down and became more cooperative.

Here one can understand the frustration felt when assistance is needed in basic care and the necessity of giving the patient time to mobilize control.

Hussian (1986) suggests the following interventions to reduce agitation and combativeness when due to memory impairment, dementia, or delirium:

Reduce the number of persons visiting or interacting with the client and make introductions at each meeting.

Maintain well-learned life patterns.

Minimize change, maintain a routine and schedule.

Provide color codes and cues to items or areas the client needs.

Move slowly into the visual field of the client and face him or her directly.

Reduce the amount of stimulation in the environment.

Ensure adequate amounts of sleep.

Use medication only when needed and not routinely.

These interventions are all based on the assumption that reducing the frustration accompanying the inability to cope with the demands of living will reduce the need to lash out at others or become combative.

Shouting   Shouting repeatedly and at a high intensity may be an expression of hostility, a bid for attention, an indication of cerebral damage, or a form of self-stimulation. The content of the shouting and the provocative elements need to be carefully considered and analyzed to determine the appropriate interventions. Incessant yelling can lead to undesirable consequences, such as retaliation, increased use of medications, and staff discomfort and, therefore, active efforts should be made to intervene rather than ignoring the behavior. When others retaliate with shouts to quiet down, it may serve as a reinforcement of the behavior, particularly if this is the only behavior that commands attention.

If the shouting appears to be accompanied by other behavior indicating discomfort, such as grimacing or rubbing, one should consider a physical cause and rule out pain, impactions, or fractures. When the shouting includes threats, the individual's anger must be addressed and provisions made for discharge of anger through exercise or contracting for a specific time and place where one can yell and vent the frustration. Staff will need to provide assurance that the right to be angry is understood and that the individual is not rejected because of it.

The use of comforting touch, such as stroking or hand-holding, often diminishes the yelling in an individual who is seeking attention or using it as a form of self-stimulation. Even in the presence of dementia, this has proved effective. Soothing music and rocking in a rocking chair have also been useful in some of these cases. Hussian (1986) suggests that shouting may be in response to sensory stimuli that create bewilderment and that wearing earmuffs may be sufficient to reduce the environmental overload. However, earphones and music might be even more useful.

Repressed Anger   Smoldering anger and resentment may be difficult to detect or diminish because the individual seldom expresses it directly. Indications that submerged anger may be present can be seen in a pattern of complaints or jealousies that seem directed toward specific persons or situations. Weber and McCall (1987, pp. 42–43) cite the case of Mrs. R., who frequently "accidentally" bumped her roommate or broke her things.

> With careful observation it was noted that these episodes occurred more frequently after the roommate had visitors. Mrs. R. also complained about the visitors' noise and criticized various things they said and did. It became apparent that Mrs. R. was jealous of the attention her roommate received as she had no visitors of her own. Relationships with her own relatives had always been poor and punctuated with quarrels and vendettas. Staff discussed her situation and realized that intepersonal relationships may have always been problematic for Mrs. R. As they were unable to provide her a private room, they transferred her to a room in which the other resident was noncommunicative and had no visitors. One staff member volunteered to spend time each day with Mrs. R. to talk about her feelings of loneliness, anger, isolation, and resentment. It was also decided that increasing her participation in energy-requiring activities that would allow her physical expression of some of the pent-up anger might be useful. Though Mrs. R. was unable to express her feelings verbally, the episodes of unintentional bumping and breaking things ceased.

Unfortunately, there are few activities in institutions designed specifically for the venting of frustration and anger yet the need is often apparent. In the community, and with youthful energy, one can smash a tennis ball, hit a golf ball, court exhaustion in racquet ball, or run. Creative efforts of staff may be necessary to develop alternative activities, suitable for the aged, to express pent-up frustration. The following activities have been used effectively:

Blanket ball bouncing. This is accomplished by several residents holding the edges of a blanket and bouncing a ball to each other by manipulating the blanket.

Throwing yarn balls. This is a means of symbolically connecting people as they hold the yarn but throw the ball to another person.
Squashing clay or dough.
Yelling sessions. These are conducted in concert and have the additional advantage of aerating the lungs.
Bowling night. Conducted in a hall with plastic pins.

Other adaptations of physically expressive activities can be identified as staff consider the needs and capabilities of residents.

Boredom

Though boredom may seldom be identified as the cause of behavioral problems or emotional outbursts, it may be more prevalent in long-term care settings than caregivers are willing to admit. It may cause disruptive actions for the sake of stimulating a response. It may cause challenges to the staff and provocative behaviors for the sake of attention. In the case of Mr. O., it stimulated attempts to bolt the facility (see the discussion in the section related to wanderers). The NANDA nursing diagnoses have identified Diversional Activity Deficit as a major nursing problem. It is rarely seriously addressed. Yet, caregivers have long recognized that the challenge of mastery in new situations is fundamental to human growth and development. In late life, situations that are new and challenging are rare at best. A long lived individual has confronted most of the real human problems that occur. If there is no stimulation, life becomes a matter of bodily survival and spiritual apathy. The old triumvirate of body, mind, and spirit are essential to humanity. Somehow, in the dedication to the technology of preserving the body, caregivers have often lost sight of the even more important significance of preserving the mind and the spirit.

What can be done to present new challenges and opportunities for growth in an institutional situation? The possibilities are provocative. Can caregivers bring the strengths of the individual to the community while recognizing their disabilities? Can caregivers bring the community to the institution while dealing with the possibility of unrealistic expectations? The solutions are not easy or readily apparent, but, not two decades ago, mainstreaming the disabled child was an outrageous idea. Can caregivers begin to think in terms of "mainstreaming" the disabled elder? Can caregivers adapt institutions to human needs in addition to survival needs? If caregivers cannot, perhaps the question of survival is moot and meaningless.

Confusion

Confusion is by far the most frequent observable symptom of distress of physical or emotional origin encountered in the aged. It ranges on a continuum from fleeting, mild disorientation (often due to Transient Ischemic Attacks (TIAs) to the profound mental deterioration of advanced Alzheimer's disease. Along the continuum, one finds confusion due to deprivation, over and understimulation, physiologic imbalance, metabolic disorders, disease processes, loss of meaning, and poor sleep processes. The following material provides a list of Psychiatric Nursing Diagnoses (PNDs) most commonly applicable in confused states.

PSYCHIATRIC NURSING DIAGNOSES RELATED TO CONFUSION

Individual, Biologic
  Hypotension
  Constipation (Impaction)
  Pain
  Dehydration
  Malnutrition
  Adverse drug reaction
  Sensory/perceptual impairment
Individual, Behavioral
  Sleep disturbances
  Agitation
  Regression
  Withdrawal/isolation
  Confabulation
  Disengagement
  Substance abuse
Individual, Emotional
  Altered level of responsiveness
  Impaired memory and intellectual function
  Impaired thought processes
  Impaired attention and orientation
Interpersonal, Identity
  Disengagement/depersonalization
Interpersonal, Stress
  Acute loss
  Resource deficits
  Routine disruption

> Interpersonal, Information Processing
>   Perception
> Interpersonal, Role Structuring
>   Role loss
> Interpersonal, Affiliation
>   Diminished social supports
> Community, Aggregate
>   Institutionalization
>   Homelessness
>   Neglect/inadequate resources

In addition to the assessment and diagnoses noted above, it is important to assess the *pattern* of confusion in an elder and the purpose it may fill. The importance of this assessment lies in devising more sentient modes of coping that will not garner the dehumanizing feedback engendered by confused thoughts and behaviors.

Wolanin and Phillips' (1981) *Confusion: Prevention and Care* is a classic and invaluable text for staff working with the confused aged in any setting. As is well known, the "early warning sign" of many disorders is confusion. Caregivers have long been aware of this and have attempted to institute rapid assessment and intervention when confusion becomes apparent.

In some cases, caregivers may find it fruitful to address their efforts toward an analysis of the human need or secondary gain arising from the confusion. Caregivers may then address the problem in a more straightforward and healthy manner. See Figure 5.1.

An example from Olga illustrates the point nicely.

Olga, a lady of regal appearance, was 76 years old and had resided in a nursing home since the death of her husband, who had been her caregiver. She was a lady of great pride and was dubbed "the duchess" by facility staff. She had indeed been a lady of high social status in her native country of Germany from which she had emigrated in 1940 . . . she was also a great problem-solver. Olga had some flattening of affect and some periods when her memory was blurred, but she was usually quite lucid. During one of my visits to the facility, she seemed almost stuporous and extremely confused. When the staff nurse left the room, Olga murmured to me, "This is the only way to get people to leave you alone around here."

I doubt any of us really comprehend the psychic pain and exhaustion contingent upon continuous loss of privacy. Many of the behaviors caregivers judge to be aberrant may, in fact, be adaptive mechanisms that serve the individual well to survive a bizarre situation. In other

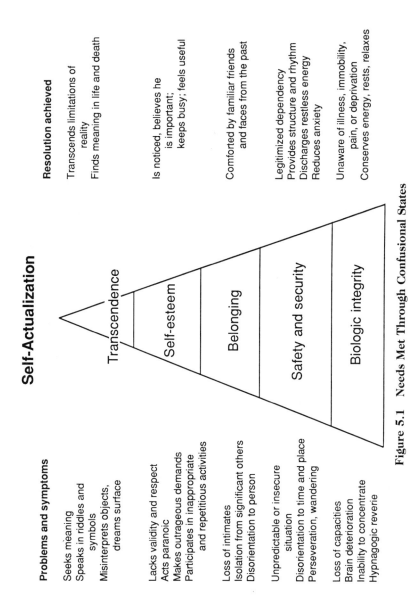

Self-Actualization

Problems and symptoms		Resolution achieved

Seeks meaning
Speaks in riddles and
  symbols
Misinterprets objects,
  dreams surface
	Transcendence	Transcends limitations of
		  reality
		Finds meaning in life and death

Lacks validity and respect
Acts paranoic
Makes outrageous demands
Participates in inappropriate
  and repetitious activities
	Self-esteem	Is noticed, believes he
		  is important;
		  keeps busy; feels useful

Loss of intimates Isolation from significant others Disorientation to person	Belonging	Comforted by familiar friends and faces from the past
Unpredictable or insecure situation Disorientation to time and place Perseveration, wandering	Safety and security	Legitimized dependency Provides structure and rhythm Discharges restless energy Reduces anxiety
Loss of capacities Brain deterioration Inability to concentrate Hypnagogic reverie	Biologic integrity	Unaware of illness, immobility, pain, or deprivation Conserves energy, rests, relaxes

Figure 5.1 Needs Met Through Confusional States

Source: From P. Ebersole & P. Hess. (1985). *Toward Healthy Aging: Human Needs and Nursing Response*, 2nd Ed. St. Louis; C. V. Mosby.

words, the situation may be the problem and the individual adaptation may be quite appropriate for the conditions.

Gillies (1986, pp. 257–261) has summarized some occurrences that affect memory and produce varying degrees of confusion (see below).

COMMON CAUSES OF CONFUSION

Circulatory problems
Toxins
Trauma
Infections
Endocrine imbalance
Nutritional deficits
Sensorial/perceptual loss
Neurotransmitter imbalances
    Dopaminergic
    Cholinergic
    Adrenergic
Cerebral nerve cell degeneration
Cerebrovascular accidents
Shortened attention span
Decreased motivation
Lack of exposure to new information
Lack of opportunity to use new information
Inadequate rehearsal of meaningful material
Selective forgetting to cope with threats

To properly assess the cause of confusion, Gillies (1986) recommends:

Detailed health history
Complete physical
Appropriate cognitive testing
    Face-Hand test (Fink, Green, & Bender, 1952)
    Mini-Mental State (Folstein, 1975)
    Misplaced Objects (Crook, Ferris, & McCarthy, 1979)
    Mental Status Questionnaire (Kahn-Goldfarb, 1960)
    Fromaje (Libow, 1977)

Astute observation
Mood
Dryness of skin, scantiness of hair
Condition of nails and buccal mucosa

While the purpose of this text is not designed to present all of the
assessment tools that are particularly useful with aged individuals,
caregivers may check the appendices for suggested assessment tools
that are useful. I would also recommend consulting the text by Kane
and Kane (1981) and Gallo et al. (1988) regarding assessment of the
elderly. Rapid diagnosis and reversal of conditions is extremely important to avoid irreversible brain damage.

Sundowners   *Sundowners* demonstrate a particular type of confusion. Most health care personnel are familiar with this problem.
Individuals who seem quite able to negotiate the environment in the
daylight hours become confused and disoriented in late afternoon. It
has usually been assumed that diurnal biorhythms of individuals in
tenuous physiologic homeostatic balance are partially responsible for
this disorder. Increased circulating cortisol levels in late afternoon
slightly amplify environmental awareness. The physiologically fragile
may not be able to integrate the sensations into coherent perceptual
fields. To compensate, a quieter environment with better lighting and
fewer demands upon the patient may be beneficial.

Evans (1987) has studied persons who exhibit "sundowners" syndrome. She found that the incidence was higher in demented persons.
In addition, those persons who had experienced several major changes
within the previous six months, whether with underlying dementia or
not, were those most prone to exhibit late afternoon and evening
confusion. Consistent statistical significance amplified the importance
of these data. It appeared that an increased stress response in individuals marginally able to adapt produced confusion. Caregivers could
easily correlate this finding with biorhythmic theories as we now
know how ongoing stress raises cortisol levels and disrupts the deli-
cate mechanisms of the body.

Suggestions for interventions that seemed most helpful in alleviating the syndrome were to increase lighting in areas that are poorly lit
and to restore as much order and predictability in the environment as
possible. Given the nature of institutions in the late afternoon when
shift changes occur, meals are prepared, visitors are beginning to
arrive, and the ever present intercom is speaking from the ceiling, it is
small wonder that vulnerable persons become confused. Though I
have not known of any facility eliminating the use of the intercom,

with present day technology it seems quite possible that each staff member could carry his/her own beeper.

In some situations, disorientation may be precipitated by deeper needs that are not recognized consciously. The individual who continually mistakes caregivers for relatives who are no longer living or who do not visit may be attempting to compensate for the absence of significant others. In cases of extreme loneliness, as in the case of Admiral Byrd (1938) at the South Pole, individuals may even hallucinate to invent the presence of companions so sorely needed. For the caregiver, orienting the person by stating identity is important but it is even more important to talk about the loneliness and the need for familiar faces and acquaintances.

> Mr. J. was approximately 75 years old. He was brought to the hospital because he was found wandering in a dazed manner down a main highway in the suburbs. He was unable to give a coherent history when he was admitted to the community mental health center, but some of his needs and past soon became apparent as he frequently approached staff asking where he could find the girls. He also frequently complained about the service in this hotel. In his confusion, he regressed to old and familiar patterns and needs. When this occurs, it may be helpful to matter-of-factly discuss how difficult it is to be in the hospital but that as he (Mr. J.) improves, he can return to his hotel and the girls. In many cases, of course, return to the previous life style may not be possible. Then, it is most helpful to focus on feelings surrounding the losses and the grief process. In addition, it is important for staff to separate their own life style from that of the patient who may have entirely different values and expectations.

Mental Status Assessment   The most commonly used cursory assessment of mental status is the Kahn and Goldfarb (1970) Mental Status Questionnaire (see Table 5.3). Although this questionnaire lacks sophistication, if used in a nonthreatening situation and replicated several times, its reliability is good.

When using the Mental Status Questionnaire, it is important to weave the questions into the context of conversation to ease the anxiety one feels when being questioned. The test should be given in a comfortable atmosphere by a caregiver with whom the client feels comfortable. Environmental cues must be available in the setting if the client is to be expected to remember dates, etc. The test should be given two or three times if the responses are not accurate. In such cases, it may be useful to give the test at another time of day or in another setting.

Promoting Self-Care in the Confused   The following suggestions of how to teach and promote self-care in the confused or cognitively impaired elder should be useful to caregivers, even prior to identifying the cause of symptom(s).

TABLE 5.3   Mental Status Questionnaire

Where are we now? (orientation to place)
Where is this place located? (orientation to place)
What month is it? (time orientation)
What day of the month is it? (time orientation)
What year is it? (time orientation)
How old are you? (memory)
When is your birthday? (memory)
Where were you born? (memory)
Who is the President of the United States? (general information and memory)
Who was President before him? (general information and memory)

Scoring: 0–2 errors, none or mild impairment
3–6 errors, moderate impairment
6–8 errors, advanced impairment
8–10 errors, severe brain dysfunction
Source: Kahn and Goldfarb (1970).

- Promote consistency and predictability in expectations.
- Make labels and environmental cues clearly visible.
- Speak clearly in language the individual can comprehend.
- Repeat necessary instructions in two or three ways within 10 or 15 minutes.
- Have personal mementoes visible.
- Provide clocks, calendars, and newspapers.
- Make selective use of radio and TV.
- Provide mild exercise to stimulate circulation.

Integrative therapy has also been suggested as a means to assist confused persons (Gillies, 1986). Specific instructions include:

- Activation of thought processes through appealing to more than one sensory mode; e.g., sight and sound, seek response, incorporate familiar patterns.
- Motivation of individual by emphasis on value of the action in promoting independence of the patient.
- Rehabilitation by identification and repair of specific cognitive deficits, encouraging individual to talk self through the required steps, placing items in places where they will be easily found or identified.
- Grouping items for magnification of stimuli.
- Modifying the environment to maximize ability.

An example may demonstrate these points. When a confused elder has difficulty selecting appropriate clothes and dressing, it would be useful to put a picture of clothing on the closet door that would show an individual in shoes, stockings, dress or shirt, and pants. The elder can then be taken to the closet where clothes will be identified and each step in dressing discussed. For example, the caregiver could say, "Put on underwear first, then dress, then stockings and shoes. Now, let's go through the steps and you repeat them with me." In addition, it may be helpful to list each step on a card to be kept on the closet door. It will also be important to reinforce the importance of selecting her own clothes and dressing herself. In this respect, the caregiver could say, "You look very nice when you are dressed and it shows that you are able to do things for yourself." "I know you want to select a special dress for your granddaughter's visit." "Let's decide which dress you will wear and place it on the end of the rack so you will find it easily this afternoon." Later, she may need assistance to dress for the visit. Prior to going to meet her visitor, she should be taken to a full length mirror and told how nice she looks. It may be useful to also rehearse some of the things she may want to talk about with her granddaughter.

Cognitive mapping is another orientation strategy that is sometimes useful for the confused. Orienting individuals to the general building layout and particular areas of importance may need to be done repeatedly. Unique posters, signposts, colored doors, photographs, all provide confirmation of individuality and may assist a person to find his or her room, the dining room, recreation room, and office.

In some cases, buddy systems have been formed in which the inherent strengths and deficits of two confused persons are matched. Occasionally, this occurs spontaneously but, if not, it could be encouraged. For example, if John tends to have difficulty finding his room and Dan has trouble remembering to go to meals, they may assist each other. Staff may need to promote and reinforce how they can help each other. Each will feel better about himself if he is able to help the other.

In one facility, it was noted that Harvey always tended to walk out of his room, turn right and toward the exit. By recognizing this pattern and changing his room so that a right turn led him to the lounge area, his tendency to wander outside was abated. Undoubtedly, past patterns had something to do with his penchant to make a right turn whenever leaving his room. Alert staff were able to realize his style and intervene effectively. The orientation guidelines below are generally useful when working with confused elders.

ORIENTATION GUIDELINES FOR WORKING
WITH CONFUSED ELDERLY

Add as many visual cues to the setting as you can. When vision is impaired, heavy reliance on consistent auditory input is essential. Check hearing aids and eyeglasses for effective function.

Make the environment as predictable as possible by anticipatory planning, printed schedules, and a safe, routine schedule. When changes must be made, introduce them slowly and rehearse expected performance with the individual involved.

Insist on a thorough physical and neuro examination to rule out organic bases of confusion. Remember that too many intrusive or diagnostic procedures in a short time will increase confusion.

Assess the stresses experienced recently and within the last two years.

A lack of stimulation or an overload of changes may both result in confusion. If sensory deprivation or lack of stimulation is the problem, add color, texture, flavor, and noncompetitive activity to the daily schedule. If an overload of new expectations and adaptations have occurred, then environmental stability, reduced expectations, rest, and continuity of supportive personnel is essential.

When confusion is extensive and organically based, reduce expectations to those that can be accomplished and give consistent, immediate praise for any degree of success. This must be done by all staff and long-term, consistent efforts are essential.

No matter what degree of confusion prevails, individuals remain sensitive to warm affect and caring gestures. A relationship that conveys the value of each human regardless of functional capacity is of the utmost importance. Recovery may not be realistic, but caring in the presence of deterioration and decline is high level nursing.

Finally, when working with individuals whose ability to give accurate feedback and warm gratitude is impaired, the caregiver may develop a solid personal peer suppport system. Those who understand the disappointments and struggles are in the best position to listen to each other. Sharing feelings, anger, exasperation, and humor allows the caregiver to continue in a very difficult task.

Crying

Crying or moaning frequently can be an irritant and lead to the rejection of the patient who engages in this behavior. If the impetus for the emotion is a bid for attention, then the behavior is exacerbated by rejection. It is important to attempt to identify the source of the pain and alleviate that before there are negative repercussions. Cuizon-Saiz (1988) provides an example illustrative of the above comments.

> Mrs. Q., a mildly demented patient, newly admitted to a long-term care facility, cried a lot and wanted to go home. This was recognized as a necessary grief reaction related to the relocation and unfamiliar environment. A companion with whom Mrs. Q. had lived brought in her favorite items and pictures to provide some continuity and maintenance of self-concept. In addition, the companion alerted the staff to memories which Mrs. Q. enjoyed discussing. The crying and compulsive requests to go home abated over time. Her companion remained a reliable friend and connection with the community and her home.

When an individual has no significant relationships the "Adopt-a-Resident" program may provide a means of developing one. Hillhaven Corporation originated this program in which each employee within the facilities is encouraged to develop an ongoing relationship with an elder who has no family or friends (see discussion on p. 9). This has made a significant difference in the adjustment reaction of some patients.

When crying or moaning seems to be a method of communication used by a nonverbal patient, it must be dealt with in that manner. Addressing the communication directly is often helpful. For example, the caregiver may respond by saying, "I know you are feeling unhappy and there are many reasons why you should. I will try to help." After checking basic comfort, positioning, thirst, and hunger, it may be helpful to provide soothing music and a plush animal for the patient to hold. Sometimes quietly holding hands or stroking may abate the crying and moaning. At times, another patient may be enlisted to sit and hold hands with the individual who is discontent.

Labile emotions following a stroke often result in unprecipitated or uncontrollable crying. For example, Violet would often cry during the remotivation group though she clearly enjoyed participating. Other group members were initially upset and thought perhaps they had done something to cause her unhappiness. The group leader said in a matter-of-fact manner, "I know you don't want to cry, Violet, but that is a result of your stroke and you will not do that as you get better." After this had occurred a few times, Violet would say, "I really don't want to cry but I know I can't help it right now."

COMMUNICATING WITH THE STROKE (CVA) PATIENT

While stroke rehabilitation is not the focus of this text, the resulting emotional reactions and physical limitations evident as an aftermath of stroke do produce behavioral management challenges and communication problems. Sine (1986) has provided excellent guidelines that are clear and applicable for dealing with lateralized stroke limitations (see Table 5.4). Such guidelines are useful in determining methods of reaching out in understanding to those patients.

As the majority of strokes affect only one side of the brain and the opposing side of the body (unilateral), this means most stroke patients have a predictable set of deficits. It is important that caregivers are familiar with these in order to develop appropriate expectations and patient goals and to avoid unnecessary patient and staff frustration. There are distinct behavioral differences between persons with right- and left-sided stroke lesions. The most striking facet of the right hemiparetic (left-hemisphere brain damage) is the inability to process symbols. This may lead to bizarre behavior but when a skill is learned there is good retention. In addition, the ability to maintain attention while learning is good though depression may be a limiting factor and severely impede rehabilitation. Left hemiparesis, on the other hand, is characterized by extreme inattention, neglect, and unawareness of the afflicted side of the body, and intact but monotone speech. Depression is less pervasive but there may be agitation and hallucinatory activity.

Rehabilitation is geared to learning of desired functions designed appropriate to the intact hemisphere's abilities. The traditional stroke program treats patients with right and left hemiplegia in much the same manner. A "lateralized stroke program," such as referred to here, is devised to deal with cognitive deficits and discrepancies and to take advantage of residual capacities (see Table 5.4).

General guidelines for stroke rehabilitation include the following:

Instructional materials must be in a format acceptable to the person's intact perceptual and intellectual capacity.
Person must be taught to use complementary functions to compensate for deficits.
Verbal instructions should be kept to a minimum to avoid overload and distraction.

TABLE 5.4   The Lateralized Stroke Program

Guidelines for Left Hemiplegia	Rationale
1. Present material on the right side. Objects to be worked on should be presented singly. Nothing that may be distracting should be further to the right of the object to which attention is to be directed.	1. Each hemisphere directs attention towards the opposite visual field. A hemispheric lesion disturbs the normal balance. The normal hemisphere, uninhibited by the damaged hemisphere, directs attention to the opposite side. The effect is of "neglect" or "agnosia" for the side of the hemiplegia, created by a biasing of attention to the contralateral side.
2. Verbal instructions should be put simply and briefly.	2. Verbal input may heighten left hemispheric activity, thereby increasing contralateral biasing of attention.
3. Work areas should be quiet with a minimum of distraction.	3. The left hemisphere is more easily alerted than the right, but habituates more rapidly. The effect is of easy distractibility and short attention span.
4. Material should be broken into small steps, then presented in logical sequence.	4. The left hemisphere utilizes sequential logistic learning.
5. Encourage verbal self-cuing to facilitate focusing and training, and particularly to compensate for spatial ability deficits and hemi-inattention.	5. The linguistic mode is the complementary mode to right hemispheric spatial superiority. It is an extremely versatile mode capable of compensating for numerous cognitive deficits.
6. Pictures are a poor learning aid.	6. The left hemisphere has poor ability to recognize and synthesize figures.
7. Do not accept the patient's assertions of adequate function.	7. Left hemiplegics often react with denial to their disability.
8. Despite the patient's reasonable verbal assurances of good judgment and concern for his personal safety, rely on observation to determine his level of activity.	8. Patients with left hemiplegia tend to demonstrate poor judgment, impulsive behavior, and confabulation.
9. No attempt should be made to confirm learning by copying or constructing pictures.	9. Right hemispheric lesions produce spatial agnosias. Such practices are likely to be unrewarding.
10. Facial expressions of approval or disapproval are not to be relied upon as "reinforcers."	10. The left hemisphere recognizes facial expression poorly. The lack of patient response may be interpreted as "poor motivation."
11. "Music room" listening as an activity is apt to be a poor reinforcer.	11. Pitch appreciation is a right hemisphere function.

(continued)

TABLE 5.4   (continued)

Guidelines for Right Hemiplegia	Rationale
1. Use verbal communication only when you are sure it is completely understood: if it is not, cease use of speech altogether.	1. Use of poorly understood speech can be distracting and may defer the use of other methods of communication. Adequate communication should not be sacrificed in hopes of providing speech therapy.
2. Use the *real* situation for a functional activity. If this is not practical, use simulated situations, pantomime, and gestures in that order.	2. The right brain best appreciates the reality in contradistinction to symbolic reconstruction such as speech, reading, mathematics, and gesture.
3. The right hemiplegic can benefit from prolonged intermittent instruction; he may benefit if allowed to remain in therapy and observe other patients' activities.	3. The right hemisphere maintains its ability to "alert" over a prolonged period. It may be expected to learn from observation.
4. Use facial expression freely to express approval, disapproval, humor, etc.	4. The right hemisphere is superior in recognition of facial expression.
5. Present material as a whole: different parts may then be gone over separately and reiterated.	5. The right hemisphere learns best in context and is able to synthesize parts.
6. Position material so it is presented from the left side.	6. The right hemiplegic has contralateral biasing of attention although it is not as well recognized nor as troublesome as it is in left hemiplegia (see left hemiplegic guidelines). It may be that the right hemiplegic compensates with his ability to synthesize whereas the same loss compounds the problem of the left hemiplegic.
7. The patient may enjoy music, singing, and playing musical instruments.	7. The right hemisphere is superior in appreciation of pitch.

From *Basic Rehabilitation Techniques* by R. D. Sine, J. D. Holcomb, R. E. Roush, S. D. Liss, and G. B. Wilson, Boulder, CO: Aspen Publications.

The first principle seems self-evident. No one attempts to teach the blind using written material yet it is easy to find examples of health care professionals giving verbal instructions to the severely aphasic patient or presenting diagrams to the spatially deficient left hemiplegic.

If caregivers draw on residual abilities and do not dwell on deficits, training will proceed quickly. The person with a right hemiplegic upper extremity deficit may be taught to accomplish activities of daily living with the intact arm and may again reach full independence.

Such training given early may also avoid much of the depression and preoccupation with the hemiplegic arm so often seen in stroke patients.

Application of these principles to cognitive losses is more subtle. The left hemiplegic's loss of spatial ability must be compensated by verbal cueing. Thus, these individuals must be "talked" through space. For example, he may learn to tell himself the way back to his room or the steps to putting on his clothing.

The right hemiplegic may be able to understand facial expressions and gestures in a way that will compensate for receptive aphasia. Response to body language cues may be so effective that family and other caregivers may believe the aphasic understands what is said.

In reflecting on the subtleties of caring for the person with residual stroke damage, the principle of focusing on strengths rather than losses is singularly important. In addition, according to Sine (1986), the hemiplegic functional limitations concurrent with stroke are not as devastating as the manner in which the individual is treated by friends, family, and caregivers. Frequently, there is subtle or even gross evidence of dehumanization apparent in the quality of interactions emanating from those in the environment of the stroke victim, often because of inadequate understanding of capacities. Some of the following guidelines may prove useful in gearing expectations to residual capacities.

PARTICULAR INCAPACITIES DUE TO
UNILATERAL STROKES

Left-sided lesions interfere with symbolic conceptualization.

Pictures and objects may be as difficult to comprehend as the spoken or written word.

Symbolic content of gestures may not be understood.

Much speech relearning takes place in the right hemisphere.

Musical pitch and harmony are left-sided functions but rhythm is right hemispheric.

Left hemisphere alerts one to attention but tires quickly; right hemisphere maintains more sustained attention.

Perseveration is not a function of the injured portion of the brain, but is a function of an intact portion of the brain attempting to compensate.

Right brain is generally positive in emotional response while left brain is emotionally negative in outlook.

> Left brain damage may appear as agitation or depression whereas right brain damage will be seen as lack of emotionality or denial.
> Right brain is thought to be responsible for the inflection, timbre, and emotional aspects of speech.

As is indicated above, communicating with some stroke patients may present special difficulties. Staff may try numerous ways to reach an individual patient before identifying the most effective, however.

PERSEVERATIVE COMMUNICATION

One of the greatest challenges to gerontologic nurses is to establish rapport and perceive a meaning in the perseverative babblings of a severely regressed old person. Indeed, it is so grating on the nerves of others that the treatment of the environment is of more concern than the individual. Thus, reliance on psychotropics for control are commonplace. Unfortunately, psychotropics are often of little help as they increase the disoriented person's difficulty. Zachow (1984) is the first individual to report successful strategies for reaching such an individual (Helen), and establishing meaning. First, and of utmost importance, Zachow would move close, use reassuring touch, and speak Helen's name. In addition to relying on the hope that Helen would recognize her own name filtering through her perceptual haze, Zachow knew the healing value of music, relaxation, and validation. She used all these strategies methodically, consistently, and with care to avoid overload. She found that touch and Largo Baroque instrumental music seemed to reach Helen and reestablish her fragmented rhythmicity of sound. After eight weeks of interaction and multiple sensory approaches, Helen was able to express herself understandably and with gratitude. Whether the strategies, the caring, or both were the ingredients that reached Helen is unclear. However, caregivers do know that certain people assumed unreachable may not be.

SEXUAL ACTING OUT

Sexual acting out in an institution may be difficult to manage. Yet it is apparent that the expression, however inappropriate, is one of the most basic human needs. Depending upon the frequency and importance of sexual activity prior to institutionalization, the deprivation of opportunities for sexual expression can be deeply disturbing and significant. There are other needs that may also be expressed through sexually provocative behavior. These behaviors may indicate any of the following: an awareness of, and fight against, the mental and physical changes of aging; the loss of others' recognition of or response to sexual identity and the attempts of the individual to retain it; deprivation of touch and affectional gestures; an attempt to express anger and to distance people; to combat depression and low self-esteem; an attempt to compensate for the loss of a companion. To effectively intervene, caregivers must attempt to discover the meaning of the behavior by a nonjudgmental discussion with the individual.

As mentioned earlier in the text, masturbation and sexual exhibition are particularly difficult for some staff to manage. However, the caregiver must not fail to recognize the probability of personal distortion or preconception when intervening here. No doubt, such recognition is difficult but necessary.

Masturbation is not inherently wrong. It is seen as inappropriate because it occurs in the wrong place. Assessment, therefore, should include environmental variables that contribute to the exhibition of the sexual behavior, such as the location of the occurrence, the recipient, and any identifiable antecedents (Hussian, 1986). The behavior may occur because, in the past, it has been followed by positive consequences, such as orgasm or attention from others.

The following considerations should be made prior to any intervention:

Who thinks the behavior inappropriate?
Is the behavior dangerous?
Does the behavior violate the right of other patients?
Does the behavior seriously disrupt ward routine?
Is the exhibitor competent?
Does the recipient of the behavior require protection?
Is the behavior actually sexual or is there other intent?
Is the behavior itself inappropriate or only occurring at inopportune places or times?

If it is decided that a sexual behavior requires attention, it must be determined whether the behavior is due to a natural need for expression or poor inhibitory control. In the first instance, the instigator may need to be separated from the audience by a change of rooms or wards. Staff must act quickly to protect clients who are incapable of providing consent to a sexual encounter.

When inhibitory control is impaired due to stroke or dementia, the sexual gestures are usually brief and not actual attempts to achieve sexual gratification. They may be bothersome but difficult to control. For example, an aged man residing in a nursing home would frequently grab the breast of a staff person or other patient. The behavior could not be reasoned out of existence but could only be dealt with firmly after the fact. Most staff had experienced similar episodes when they were adolescent but were particularly affronted by the old man's advances. Staff discussed their feelings and decided that removing the man's hand and telling him calmly that they would not allow that was the best way to handle it. They also agreed that they should not avoid him but might sit with him and hold his hand to show their acceptance of him and to meet some of his need for contact with females.

In cases where a demented patient masturbates, strips, or exposes genitals in public, Hussian (1986) found that the client's behavior could be controlled by immediately removing the client to his or her room and encouraging him or her to reach orgasm by masturbation in the privacy of the room.

In a classic article, Gochros (1972) discussed the sexual oppression of the mentally ill, the imprisoned, and the aged. Elderly widows, particularly, find their sexual rights limited, withdrawn, or unavailable. Some of the reasons for abdication of sexual rights stem from physiologic changes, untreated or overly aggressive treatment of disease conditions, social taboos, and lack of opportunities. Frequently, older patients are subjected to medical treatments that will impair or destroy their capacity for intercourse yet this aspect may never be discussed. It is as if caregivers conclude, without asking, that this is unimportant in the later years.

To deal with this subject in a more compassionate and understanding way, Genevay (1986) suggests that caregivers must first confront their own attitudes toward sexuality. This entails a reflection on family and personal sexual history and values, and an anticipation of individual aging. Particular suggestions for dealing with the objectionable behavior are provided below.

DEALING WITH BEHAVIORAL MANIFESTATIONS OF SEXUALITY

Caregivers should ask themselves, "What does this mean in the context of the patient's life?"
Imagine themselves without sex, affection, or touch.
Assume nothing about the behavior until they determine the meanings.

Talk about sexual needs as one adult to another, not as a parent. Listen without judgment.

Ask the painful questions but recognize that caregivers don't have all the answers.

Encourage discussion of past history of love and intimacy.

Establish specific guidelines for appropriate expression of the suppressed need.

Assist family to examine restrictive stereotypes they may have about elders and sexuality.

Advocate for the patient's right to sexual expressions, fantasies, sexual feelings, masturbatory activity, wish, and massage or other sensual experiences, if the patient wishes.

Risk relating in affectional ways and encourage gestures of affection and caring.

Adapted from Genevay (1986)

Some of the complexities of dealing with the issues of sexuality lie in the degree of responsibility caregivers feel for those individuals who no longer have the capacity for sound judgment related to sexual encounters. As one nurse told me, "In our institution we make opportunities for consenting adults to have privacy for intercourse if they wish. The problem is that I'm not sure Grace is capable of making that decision, and I would want someone to protect my mother from doing something so out of character for her." As Genevay (1986) suggests, caregivers must know their own values and not impose them on others yet caregivers must also try to understand the genuine wishes of those under their care. Perhaps caregivers must remind themselves again and again that they don't have all the answers and must rely on best judgment under the scrutiny of self-awareness. Staff meetings and discussions may be frequently necessary to explore motivations and the difficult decisions related to patient management.

WANDERING

Wandering is one of the most difficult management problems encountered in institutional settings. Each year some residents wander away from a facility and are later found injured or dead. Media attention and litigation may suggest that facility staff have been lax in allowing this to happen. Some elders are obsessed with the thought of leaving a facility and in spite of the best efforts of staff they will find a way to do so unless physically restrained.

Ambulation, in and of itself, is necessary and sufficient opportunities to do so in areas that are not hazardous are needed in institutional settings. Individuals whose life styles have included great amounts of ambulation are particularly in need of opportunities to continue this behavior. The rate or amount of ambulation may seem excessive but, if it is not inherently dangerous, it should be allowed without interference. The pattern and route of ambulation as well as the point at which it terminates are significant.

Hussian and Davis (1983) analyzed ambulatory patterns in institutionalized geriatric clients and identified four possible causes for the behavior. The patterns are as follows:

1. Akathisia-induced ambulation which is usually a result of long-term use of neuroleptics and is associated with other signs of akathisia, such as inability to sit still, repetitive movements, and other extrapyramidal symptoms. Anti-parkinsonian medication may reduce motor restlessness. Usually these persons will not do anything dangerous if made aware of the hazards.
2. Exit-seeking behavior most often exhibited in recently admitted patients on locked wards. The behavior is accompanied by statements reflecting a desire to go home. Distracting activities may be temporarily useful. Exit-seeking behavior is highly motivated and may persist until the individual finds some gratifications in the present environment that reduce the desire to leave. It may be useful to bring some significant items from the home to help the individual feel more comfortable in the unfamiliar setting.
3. Self-stimulatory behavior that takes the form of ambulation. This is often seen in advanced dementia and is associated with other stereotyped actions such as furniture rubbing, hand clapping, and repetitive vocalizations. Little has been done to deal effectively with stereotypy. Providing other forms of stimulation such as paper, cloth, or stuffed toys to manipulate may reduce the meaningless repetitive behavior. Continuous self-stimulation may indicate a lack of external sensory stimulation in the environment.
4. Modeling occurs when a severely demented client shadows an ambulator and will follow him whe:ever he or she may go. Engagement in other activities has proved useful to deter the shadowing. (Summarized from Hussian pp. 129–130, 137–138.)

Three of these patterns (1, 3, and 4) are secondary forms of wandering that are not motivated by the primary desire to achieve a goal and are, in fact, evidence of neurologic disorders. The interruption of these behaviors may cause more distress for the clients and is usually not necessary. It is also most productive to modify the environment so that the wandering is not likely to be hazardous.

Snyder, Rupprecht, Pyrek, Brekhus, and Moss (1978) published a classic study exploring this subject. In their study, they also provided a useful summary of studies to that date. Tension, inactivity, psychological conflict, environmental chaos, situational insecurity, searching (often for a significant other), and agenda behaviors were listed as distinctive causes for wandering. Recognizing those at risk of wandering and dealing with needs before they fulminate may forestall problems. Those most at risk function at lower social levels; exhibit a greater range of motion on wards; generally move about more; have a life history of motoric activity; and use walking to cope with upsetting feelings.

Snyder et al. (in Liptzin, 1986) found predictors of wandering behavior included: moving about more than others, social isolation, calling out and screaming, and some degree of dementia. Unfamiliarity with the setting did not seem to be the cause of wandering. In time/motions studies, three distinct types of wandering behaviors were identified: overtly goal-directed to searching, overtly goal-directed/industrious, and apparently non-goal-directed. Snyder et al. also suggested psychosocial factors that may influence the tendency to wander: life-long patterns of coping with stress, previous work roles, and search for security.

The environmental chaos that most frequently precedes the wandering of a resident include shift changes, noisy housekeeping, deliveries, and disorganization related to facility emergencies.

Rader, Doan, and Schwab (1985) identified and studied agenda behaviors. They found that many wanderers had a specific pattern that gave clues as to their needs. When the need was met the wandering abated. The example below illustrates their findings.

During a shift change, Mr. O.'s boredom led to his attempt to "escape" from the facility in which he had been placed. Two years previously he had suffered a severe stroke which left him paralyzed on the left side. He had hoped to live with a sister but she died and he had no alternative but placement in a nursing home. He was bored by the activities and routines. His excellent intelligence remained intact and brewed a storm of frustration. One lovely spring day, Mr. O. wheeled his chair to the front door and began screaming, "Get out of my way! I'm leaving this place." He was wheeled back to his room as he protested the entire way. One staff member recognized that the nursing home did not provide stimulation for an active mind and discussed this with Mr. O. She asked him to consider his need for physical care but also indicated her interest in helping him find a way to meet his intellectual needs. In a setting where many of the residents are demented, it is most difficult for an alert and intelligent individual to find stimulating companions. The staff member asked Mr. O. to consider ways his needs might be better met. It was finally mutually decided that he be transported to a "Great Books" discussion at the local library each week, that he conduct a current affairs group discussion in the facility each week, and that he would teach English language skills to staff for whom English was a second language. Mr. O. was a retired school teacher and these solutions were appropriate to his abilities.

Unfortunately, too often, major physical disabilities are construed as mental impairments as well.

Injury and the inability to return to the facility are the primary concerns regarding wanderers. Urban facilities must be particularly concerned about the environmental hazards one might encounter outside the institution. Considering the number of homeless elders on the streets of large cities, it is unlikely that citizens will pay much attention or offer assistance to someone who seems confused or aimlessly wandering.

Interventions suggested to prevent wandering include the following:

Music, exercise groups, and dances to provide opportunities to move in an integrated manner.
Memory development.
Mental maps of the area to increase orientation.
Massage to reduce generalized tension.
Imagery exercises to take mental trips to places one enjoyed.
Nature walks outside the facility to provide relief from the institutional setting.
Visit places of importance such as work sites and homes.

Most important, upon admission the patient and family should discuss the hazards of wandering versus the hazards of restraints or confinement and make a deliberate decision about when and if an individual should be restricted. One nursing home confers with patient and family regarding their wishes and assumption of responsibility if they decide against restraints (Kaufmann, Margaret Wagner House, Cleveland). For wanderers, electronic ankle bracelets embedded in plastic, for comfort and ease of bathing, can be put on. Should the wanderer pass through an exit, the bracelets will activate alarms installed there. A lighted panel alerts staff to the exit one has crossed. This system allows others to enter and leave the facility at will and eliminates the need for locked exits. The system, Secure Care, designed by Fennelly (see resources) is successful and somewhat costly but may be well worth the investment. There are other electronic tracking devices that are being used to follow the wanderings of some individuals.

One veterans' home uses bright colored shirts and blouses to identify individuals that the staff must watch closely to prevent wandering (WestSide Veterans Administration Medical Center, Chicago). Another home uses bells on shoes. It is doubtful that this is very useful and is too reminiscent of toddlers to be acceptable.

A particularly appealing method of dealing with the wandering patient is to form a buddy system with an individual who is willing and able to provide companionship for varying periods and can account for the patient's presence. This might increase the socialization of each, protect the wanderer, and enhance the ego of the "buddy." The "buddy" must not be coerced into such an arrangement, however. Sometimes these have formed spontaneously.

Cuizon-Saiz (1988) found maintaining eye contact and pleasant chatter was most effective when dealing with a demented old lady who repeatedly wandered away during personal care. It seemed the voice and eye contact provided a focus for her attention, somewhat like a radar beam, that kept her on course. Perhaps the personal attention also filled the empty restlessness that activated her wandering.

Rader, Doan, and Schwab (1985) investigated ways of dealing with wandering behavior that accompanies restlessness caused by anxiety and dementia. Because wandering so often is precedent to restriction and institutionalization, it is an important issue to resolve, if possible. Currently, the tendency is to reorient the confused individuals to the present and attempt in various ways to restrict their wandering. Unfortunately, this is not a particularly effective intervention, usually leaving the caregiver and patient both frustrated. Rader, Doan, and Schwab, however, report success in dealing with the behavior as a subverted message of loneliness, separation, and unmet need. In this respect, the confused individual is taking steps, however ineffective, to alleviate these feelings. Among those elders included in their study, three needs predominated: (1) the need to be with people who provided comfort and security; (2) the search for relief; and (3) the need to be needed. To meet these needs caregivers would talk about the patient's feelings and the needs and find a way for the patient to express them within the setting. Even though the patient may suffer cognitive clouding, the caregiver's tone of voice and gently guiding touch may dissuade the patient from wandering further. It was found that respecting the individual's "agenda behavior" reduced the need, saved time, and brought the patient more in touch with reality. Donat (1983) reported a similar approach as effective. In the cases he discussed, a controlled observation and analysis of wandering behavior revealed that it was not purposeless. In fact, a pattern could be clearly determined. Looking for an attractive view from a window, going to a mirror, finding a quiet place or seeking a friend were some of the speculations arising from analysis of patterns of wandering. Below are listed steps to decrease wandering as devised by Rader, Doan, and Schwab (1985, p. 198).

STEPS TO DECREASE WANDERING

Face the resident and make direct contact if this does not appear to be threatening.

Gently touch the resident's arm, shoulder, back, or waist if he or she does not move away.

Listen to what the resident is communcating verbally and nonverbally. Link this to the resident's feelings.

Identify the agenda, the resident's plan of action, and the emotional needs the agenda is expressing.

Repeat specific words or phrases from the agenda ("fix supper," "your children,") or state the need or emotion ("You need to go home?" "You're worried that your family won't be fed?").

If such repetition fails to distract the resident from leaving, accompany him or her and continue the connecting device or repeating phrases and the underlying emotions you identify.

Provide orienting information only if it calms the person. If it increases distress, stop talking about the present situation.

At intervals, redirect the resident toward the facility by suggesting, "Let's walk this way now."

If orientation and redirection fail, continue to walk, allowing the resident to control the direction but ensuring safety.

Various recommendations for managing wanderers could be categorized as rehabilitative, compensatory, or alterations in milieu and management. Rehabilitative efforts were aimed at orientation, visiting reference points in the community, providing a rigorous schedule of physical and social activities, and anxiety relief. Compensatory approaches included use of environmental cues, signs, and altering the environment to include sheltered courts and areas safe for wandering. Management changes focused on accurate observation and charting of moods, nonverbal behavior, and patterns of wandering.

Frequently, the "quick fix" is employed through the use of physical and chemical restraints. For immediate purposes, this may seem easiest but it is dehumanizing. Caregivers do not tie their children down to keep them out of danger. The Chalet Nursing Home in Yakima, Washington, mentioned in Chapter 3, has modified the entire environment and fenced in the large grounds to make wandering safe. Tub gardens are provided for each resident who wishes one, an added pleasure for those who have so little.

As previously discussed, contact with nature, while important to morale, has been little studied in relation to institutionalization. There is some conjecture that separation from the natural environment has more profound effects than caregivers currently imagine.

PASSIVITY

Powerlessness often appears as passivity and is a result of perceived lack of control over a situation and the belief that actions will not significantly effect an outcome. Gordon (1985) defines the characteristics of three levels of powerlessness:

- Severe, due to physical deterioration in spite of compliance with regimen; exhibited by apathy, depression, and verbalization of total lack of control.
- Moderate, due to erosion of identity and self-esteem; exhibited by frustration, expressed doubts about role performance, neglect of self-care, attempts to please caregivers, and dependence upon them.
- Mild, due to unfamiliar settings and uncertainty about energy for coping with requirements.

Underlying factors are related to illness, health care environment, style of interpersonal interactions, lifestyle of helplessness, and feelings of powerlessness.

Powerlessness induced by deteriorating illness in spite of the individual's best efforts to comply with the health regimen is particularly difficult to combat. It may be possible to mutually consider ways to alter the health regimen in order to increase the quality of life. Too often, caregivers think more in terms of protocol than individual need when it comes to dealing with diseases. Encouragement regarding tenacity and compliance will need to be frequently given. Focusing on the meaning of illness may bring new insights that will make the disease more tolerable.

One aged man in an acute-care unit in a hospital in California, with myriad diabetic complications and deteriorating capacities was encouraged by the discussion of his ability to compensate for many of his problems. He could accept his illness as a test of his faith and felt that he was providing an example for others in his adaptation to his limitations. He was especially interested in meeting with student nurses to help them understand the complexities of dealing with diabetes. In addition, it was determined that one of his daily irritations was insulin injections. He was given an insulin dispensing implant to alleviate one of the small irritations in his life. Since his vision was rapidly deteriorating it was important to increase availability of music that he enjoyed.

Interpersonal interactions that promote powerlessness are inherent in those interactions that are not egalitarian. Caregivers, for example, often promote powerlessness by their "good" intentions. Trying to "help" others must be examined carefully to be sure that motivations are not based on unconscious dependency needs. As the adolescent mother often sees her child as a method of playing out her own dependency needs, caregivers may look at the frail elder as an extension of themselves in later years and thus overcompensate by "giving" more than is necessary. If caregivers can remember that their best interventions may be in *refraining* from helping, they will have mastered part of the problem. Keeping a clear vision of self-determination and self-care as the highest goal for self and other may also allow the caregiver to avoid some interpersonal problems. Needless to say, patronizing attitudes easily creep in when dealing with elderly patients who appear frail and limited in options. Therefore, each caregiver must face him or herself squarely and question motives as well as means of relating to others.

Many elders in the health care system have apparently lived a lifestyle of dependence on others. Can people change when old and frail and become more independent? Is there any reason for them to do so when it appears to be easier for them and caregivers to maintain the status quo? The question may be more sensibly approached by examining the results of the dependency. Are the staff and individual finding the situation acceptable and are warm interactions apparent? Is the individual deteriorating physically due to his or her dependency? What is the nature of the dependency? What negative results are evident in the setting due to the individual's dependency? Again, perhaps staff motivations must be examined. If independence is sought for an individual purely to prove the endurance or power base of the parties involved, then it may not be a healthy avenue to pursue for the staff or patient.

Avoiding any taint of dependency promotion has been the hallmark of mental health centers and is sometimes carried to extremes. Often the grooming and physical needs of a patient are largely neglected until he or she is able to accomplish these without aid. While there is some basis to these actions (many emotionally disturbed individuals are seeking rescue and would not take the initiative to function if someone else assumed it for them) patient care must be tempered, particularly for the elderly who may need physical and emotional assistance beyond that usually provided in typical mental health centers. As greater proportions of mental health clients are older, staff will need intensive guidance and education related to elder clients' special needs. In league with these efforts, staff must also examine their own attitudes toward dependency and aging.

Slimmer, Lopez, LeSage, and Ellor (1987) studied helplessness among a group of persons in the long-term care unit of Hines Veterans Hospital in Chicago. They were interested in components of the condition, staff, and patient perceptions of helplessness. "Helplessness" was characterized by dysfunction in the areas of motivation, cognition, and affect. Patients felt they had "given up." Some nurses thought the "helpless" behaviors were motivated by the desire for attention and that, in fact, it demonstrated in a perverse way the control residents could exert. This idea deserves further attention and research. Caregivers readily accept the contrary ways of the passive/ aggressive patient as aggressive in motive if not in action. Perhaps some patients may see helplessness as their last refuge of control.

Golander (1987), using the anthropologic fieldwork approach, spent considerable time in an Israeli nursing home observing residents and concluded that there was much action going on under the guise of passivity. Most of the activity she identified focused on complexities of adjustment to nursing home reality by the physically and cognitively disabled aged. She identified four of their major concerns:

1. Protection from physical discomfort.
2. Relating to others in a way that would get their needs met.
3. Finding meaningful events in the boredom of routine.
4. Lowering their aspirations to meet their present abilities.

In this situation, Golander noticed that even the smallest actions of caregivers were carefully noted by residents, assessed, and often great significance attributed to them. In this respect, Golander's study points out several questions (listed below) that caregivers should ask of themselves.

- First, can caregivers protect individuals from discomfort if that is their great fear? If caregivers cannot, then do they take time to explain why some procedure is going to be uncomfortable?
- Second, do caregivers demonstrate that the "good patient" is the first to get their needs met?
- Third, do caregivers recognize that any small events of daily life can provide something to think about when the days are drab? Burnside (1976) noted that the fire in a facility laundry provided topics of conversation for several days.
- Fourth, how aware are caregivers that moving the seating arrangement in the dining room may carry great significance for some residents as they ponder reasons and significance?

Hess (in Ebersole & Hess, 1985) has conceptualized the "Spiral of Dependency" (Figure 5.2) that occurs when an individual seeks to meet a need but is not given recognition for his or her own problem-solving ability or decision-making power. Unfortunately, because by definition caregivers assume responsibility for and authority over elderly residents, caregivers are vulnerable to maintaining that dependency. While caregivers may be initially willing to allow elderly residents independence, as they become more and more dependent, caregivers can become annoyed and even disgusted. To counteract this, one might, in fact, develop a parallel spiral of caregiver disengagement concurrent with the increasing dependency of the client.

An example may highlight the progression of client dependency and professional withdrawal.

Mary is admitted to a nursing home following treatment for a left hemisphere CVA. She has residual damage that leaves her with right-sided weakness, expressive aphasia, and hemanopsia (½ visual field in each eye). She tries to understand what the plans for her rehabilitation may be and how long she is expected to be in the nursing home. The nurse who seems to be in charge of admitting her assesses her agitation but is unable to understand what she wants and believes it is purely a reaction to the newness of the setting and the difficulties the patient is generally experiencing. She speaks to her in a soothing voice, attempts to make her comfortable, and reassures her that she is safe and will be well cared for in the setting. Mary's agitation does not diminish and the nurse leaves to assume other duties. Upon her return later, she finds Mary trying vainly to use the telephone. Due to her deficits and apparent frustration, the telephone is removed from the room. The nurse complains that regardless of how she tries to help, Mary does not settle down and the nurse feels very

Self-Esteem, Status, and Self-Respect

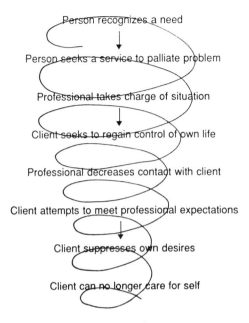

Person recognizes a need

Person seeks a service to palliate problem

Professional takes charge of situation

Client seeks to regain control of own life

Professional decreases contact with client

Client attempts to meet professional expectations

Client suppresses own desires

Client can no longer care for self

Figure 5.2   Spiral of Dependency

Developed by Patricia Hess
Source: From P. Ebersole & P. Hess. (1985). *Toward Healthy Aging: Human Needs and Nursing Response*, 2nd Ed. St. Louis; C. V. Mosby.

frustrated. When the nurse returns to the room, she finds Mary withdrawn, her face turned to the wall. Half her food has been consumed and the other half is upon the plate, untouched. Two days later Mary seems to have resigned herself to bed and refuses to exert even minimal effort toward grooming and dressing. The nurse finds herself feeling irritated at Mary's increasing helplessness and simply provides necessary care in a routine manner.

For the sake of demonstration, this example is time compressed but it is a common problem with many patients. How could this sequence of events have been turned around? The admitting nurse needs to take extra time in orienting the patient to the expectations within the setting. It is also extremely important to validate the feelings and thoughts the patient may be experiencing. In this respect the admitting nurse might say: "Mary, I know this is difficult for you when others can't understand what you need but we will try. You will begin speech therapy next week and the occupational therapist will assist you to learn ways to manage your grooming and dressing. It is important for you not to neglect your right side but to restore the lost function. The occupational therapist will help you with exercises to accomplish this. You will not be able to see food on the right side of your plate or things happening to the right side. You will need to turn your head to get a full view. We will bring you some picture cards so that you can show us things you want or need. It is going to be hard work to regain what you have lost but we will work with you to help you in accomplishing the most that you can. In the meantime, I will walk with you to the dining room and introduce you to a few of our residents."

Due to the anxiety inherent in new situations and Mary's impairments, it is doubtful that she will comprehend or remember most of what was said. Therefore, repetition will be necessary later and seeking confirmation from the patient by asking for a nod of the head if she understands. Though much information may be lost, it is important to assume the patient can understand so that maximum response will be available as she gradually becomes able to integrate it.

> Agnes provides another common example of the spiral of dependency. She is a frail, osteoporitic elderly lady who lives alone. She fell and collapsed a thoracic vertebra which produced extreme pain. Her long-time physician prescribed a strong controlled substance for pain relief and told her she must hire an attendant or move to a nursing home as it was not safe for her alone at home. Agnes was reluctant to hire an attendant as she was very frugal and took great pride in her independence but she complied with the physician's directive as she felt dependent upon him for pain control. Having never been told that alternative methods, such as hypnotism, biofeedback, or acupuncture, might provide satisfactory relief in a much healthier manner, she continued taking the strong, and addictive, medication. Because of the "helpfulness" of the attendant, the strength of the medication, the emetic effects and Agnes' frailty, she was soon totally bedridden. Family members who had not seen her in two months and had not followed the process of her deterioration were called and she was promptly placed in a nursing home.

It is quite common to retrospectively recognize this process as built into our health system in such a subtle manner caregivers hardly notice its occurrence. The roots lie in the absolute confidence many elders have traditionally placed in the judgment of their doctor. Of course, in this era of specialization, "their" doctor may be several physicians with conflicting philosophies of patient management.

DISTURBED SLEEP PATTERNS

Normal and abnormal sleep patterns in late life are frequently the cause of expressed concerns by elders. The literature disagrees but most say total sleep time normally remains constant throughout adulthood and reduced in late life. It is generally agreed that awakening for brief periods is to be expected and some persons find themselves going to bed earlier and waking earlier than when they were younger. In addition, many nap more frequently in the daytime, particularly after meals or at quiet times. Because naps do not seem to affect patterns of nighttime sleep, this need not be discouraged (Bahr & Gress, 1985).

Normal and disturbed sleep are both affected by the process of aging. Sleep disorders in the aged are more frequent and quite different from those in the young. Psychological distress is less frequently a cause of wakefulness in the aged than in the young. Sleep deprivation results in decreased concentration, drowsiness, irritability, behavioral changes, lethargy, and "micro-sleeps."

Sleep disorders in the elderly can be attributed to many factors. Changes of physiologic structure of sleep due to increasing age include decrease in the duration of "deep sleep," decreases in REM sleep, increased episodes of wakefulness, and dozing. Equally important are the somatic changes that directly or indirectly alter the course and maintenance of sleep. These include changes in respiratory and cardiovascular functions, decreases in brain perfusion, pain, discomfort, and itching. Mental changes, such as depression and varying degrees of dementia, also significantly influence sleep patterns. Contrary to most data, Spiegel (1987) found that inversion of the day–night sleep cycle in hospitalized demented patients was uncommon. However, these data need further replication and investigation. Empirically it has long been observed that demented patients seem to reverse their sleep cycles. Possibly they may be trained back to more appropriate patterns in much the same way as one trains infants to sleep at night: solid and nutritious food, warm baths, soothing lullabyes, rocking, and providing a quiet environment.

Even though sleep pattern reversal is not consistently supported in the research literature, it is a significant problem for families as well as institutional staff. Cuizon-Saiz (1988) reports that most patients with Alzheimer's disease have particular sleep difficulties in the admission adjustment period. Also empirically established is that appetite patterns may be disturbed. Alzheimer's patients are frequently hungry in the late evening, for example. As a result, offering a large snack prior to bedtime has been useful in encouraging sleep. In addition, some Alzheimer's patients fall asleep in places other than the bed. If it is not dangerous, staff should be instructed to pillow their head and cover them with blankets. In addition, patients with advanced Alzheimer's disease often find the need for narcoleptics and neuroleptics in addition to the above strategies.

Interference with sleep may stem from a number of factors:

Pathophysiologic problems such as pain, asthma, apnea, and dysp-
nea.
Misunderstanding of the sleep patterns normal to the aged.
Short-term situational life style disruptions.
Sustained and chronic stress.
Affective disorders.
Dementias.
Withdrawal from drugs or alcohol.
Hypoglycemia.
Lack of daytime activity.
Urinary frequency, incontinence, prostatitis.
Environmental stimulation at night.

Pathophysiologic sleep disorders have been given particular attention in recent years. Sleep apnea is one such disorder. An individual
with this condition stops breathing briefly, is aroused and starts
breathing again, then falls back to sleep. This cycle is repeated many
times during the night. It seems to occur almost exclusively in men
between the ages of 40 and 65 years and is accompanied by excessive
daytime drowsiness and very loud snoring at night, broken by periods
of silence. The cause of this disorder is unknown. Narcolepsy is a less
frequent disorder that is characterized by spontaneous and unpredic-
table brief episodes of daytime sleep. Unlike normal napping, these
sleep episodes are often accompanied by vivid hallucinations. This
condition usually begins before age 50.

Osis (1986) reports on particular drugs that disturb the normal
sleep patterns of the elderly. Those that are commonly taken are
particularly significant in the following ways:

Antiparkinsonians (including all those that are given to counteract
the effects of psychotropics, such as Haldol®, are associated with
a high incidence of extrapyramidal symptoms) often result in
nightmares.
Antipsychotics, particularly Navane, intensify insomnia.
Central nervous system stimulants, less commonly used for the
aged, increase the time necessary to fall asleep.
Cardiac glycosides create daytime drowsiness.
Thyroid preparations can create insomnia if blood levels are elevated.

Some interventions suggested by Osis (1986) that may be effective
in increasing residents' sleep satisfaction include:

Establishing personalized sleep rituals according to the client's preference.

Establishing a sleep–wake log for two weeks to determine patterns of sleeplessness.

Establishing a consistent time for retiring and arising.

Napping during mornings only (some studies disagree).

Practicing relaxation exercises.

Exercising daily and participating in mild exercise two hours before bedtime.

Reducing sensory input and environmental stimulation.

Avoiding drinks with caffeine throughout the day and particularly in the evening; these include coffee, tea, chocolate, and many carbonated drinks. A small alcoholic nightcap may act as a stimulant rather than a sedative.

Getting up if not asleep in 30 minutes and engaging in a quiet activity or having a snack; avoiding snacks that are hard to digest. A small glass of warm milk may help for those who do not have lactose intolerance. The benefits of L-tryptophan have not yet been proven.

Recognizing that for many, sexual activity preceded sleep and its absence may be significant.

Being sure the bed is comfortable and warm; using the bed only for sleep at night.

Hypnotics should be used for short term only; chloral hydrate remains the safest and most quickly metabolized. The effectiveness of sedatives declines after about two weeks of daily use.

As mentioned previously, plush animals may, for many reasons, be useful for sleep. Francis and Baly (1986) found that they were often held and stroked and seemed to provide an element of relaxation and comfort. They may also ease the loneliness experienced by those who have habitually had a partner in bed. It is difficult to express the precise feeling that occurs when one reaches out for the other and finds only emptiness. The "ache to hold" has not been expressed in any of the literature I have found but it is a very real physical sensation of needing someone to hold. One widow, married for 35 years, said, "Several decorative pillows and a large stuffed turtle adorn my bed. At night they are pushed to one side and the bed never seems so empty. Sometimes, I hold the turtle."

While some patients may resist going to bed and to sleep, others refuse to get up. This is often an indication of deep depression and should be treated as such. Periods of rest must be interspersed with periods of activity to the level the individual can tolerate. Other reasons people stay in bed may be due to low energy levels, incipient illness, need for privacy, or lack of incentive to interact. Cuizon-Saiz (1988) provides an appropriate example below of a resident who refused to get up.

> Mrs. R. was a tiny 84-year-old lady who liked to stay in bed. She would pull the curtains around her bed, curl up in a tight little ball, pull the covers over her head, and spend her day intermittently dozing and musing. When staff attempted to dislodge her, she would swear and try to hit them. She often missed meals and became increasingly frail. Staff recognized her right to retreat but were concerned about her physical status. They found a comfortable chair with good postural supports and enticed her to sit in it in the activity room and observe for brief periods each day. They did not push her to join in. They served her meals in the activity room as well. She seemed comfortable in the room, still dozing frequently. This routine eventually resulted in some mild interest in the activities of others around her. Though she did not participate, she would watch. Her nutrition was improved and the staff were cognizant of and gratified by her small gains. Staff discussion of her situation clarified the issues: little energy, need for discrete periods of privacy, musings that may be more gratifying than the reality, and a life pattern of being rather reclusive.

FALLS

One of the most difficult and serious problems in long-term care is falls.

Lund and Shafer (1985) demonstrated that 78% of falls in facilities studied could have been anticipated based upon physiologic problems of the patients observed. Those who were disoriented or had difficulty ambulating were at greatest risk. With this knowledge, it would be reasonable to institute special care measures to assist these persons in ambulation. Table 5.5 provides information related to patient characteristics and preventative measures. Statistics from the study cited may also be useful in preventing some falls. Forty percent of the accidents occurred between 8:00 a.m. and 4:00 p.m., 38% of patients involved in accidents had no evidence of dementia, 81% of the accidents were caused by the patient or were from unknown causes, only 2% were attributed to hazards in the environment. Sixty-three percent of the accidents occurred in the patient's room or bathroom. These statistics related to falls in the elderly were gathered during the course of one year in a facility devoted to the care of the chronic degenerative patient. One hundred seventy falls occurred among 110 patients. Other facts Lund and Shafer identified were:

Greatest number of falls occurred between 10:00 a.m. and 4:00 p.m.

TABLE 5.5 Types of Patient Falls, Patient Characteristics, and Preventative Measures

Type of fall	Patient characteristics	Prevention
I. Physiological— anticipated (78%)	Disoriented Difficulty ambulating —weak/impaired gait —poor balance —walking aids	Active prevention Provide —assistance —supervision —surveillance —well-fitting shoes
II. Physiological-unanticipated (8%)	Oriented —drop attacks —dizzy, faint —drug reaction	Active prevention Anticipate recurrence —teach patient —warn patient
III. Accidental (14%)	Normally oriented —roll out of bed —trip —slip	Passive prevention Manipulate environment —safety precautions

From Morse et al., "Characteristics of Fall-Prone Patients," *The Gerontologist*, 1987.

More men than women fell.
Seasonal variations were not noted.
45% of falls occurred while patient was walking.
29% of falls were from bed.
22% of falls were from wheelchair.
Fractures occurred in 11% and head injuries in 42% of cases.
Causes of falls could be identified in a very small number of cases.

Those at risk of falling can be identified and given special attention. The following percentages show that patients with TIAs are most likely to fall:

TIAs	60%
Vertebrobasilar syndrome	40%
Dementia	28%
Arthropathy	25%
Parkinson's disease	23%
Anxiety and depression	23%
Blindness	20%
Anemics	17%

Quite obviously, some persons had several disorders as the totals exceed 100%. Falls due to osteoporitic bone weakening may be found in men and women. Males with low levels of testosterone and hypogonadism have been found to be predisposed to osteoporosis and fractures. This suggests that osteoporosis prevention for older men may have been neglected as it has largely been considered a problem of post-menopausal women.

Johnston (1987) studied fall prevention styles of the elderly in independent living facilities. She identified three categories of fall prevention responses:

Slow watchers who watched, waited, and proceeded slowly.
Planners who avoided dangers and modified their environments.
Do nothings who predominantly did nothing to prevent a fall.

Slow watchers had the fewest falls while *planners* had significantly more. *Do nothings* were evenly distributed between the groups. One may speculate that anxiety levels of the planners may have made them more vulnerable to falling. Other factors that were significant in the predisposition to falls were: multiple medical diagnoses, polypharmacy, higher prevalence of cardiovascular and musculoskeletal disorders, and fallers had experienced more unpleasant life events in the past year than the nonfallers. Given the findings in this study, it may be advisable to construct a fall-risk profile for each frail elder upon admission to a facility.

Falls that occur because of vestibular disturbances may be prevented by postural training. Adaptive mechanisms of balance function can be stimulated by exercises and has been found to have good results in the elderly.

Consideration of the effects of drugs on proprioception and instability deserves attention. Caregivers are usually quite attuned to the drugs that create hypotension and ataxia. Frail, older persons receiving them are monitored quite well. It is also helpful to consider the rate of metabolism when a drug is being selected and always opt for the shorter acting drug. These have been shown to significantly reduce falls.

INCONTINENCE

Adult incontinence is a most dehumanizing and psychologically destructive experience. Toileting habits are established long before we have any memory of childhood events and they are thereafter taken for granted. They form a foundation for our sense of autonomy and self-control. If we lose control of these basic functions, we have profoundly altered our self-concept.

Incontinence can be a physiologically or psychologically based problem and sometimes embodies elements of both. Hess (1985b), Field (1979), and other studies have shown that incontinence often begins in the course of an acute hospitalization and the frightened and chagrined patient never returns to full continence following the first loss of control. In the unfamiliar setting of a hospital, under heavy medication, depleted by illness, and with the bed siderails raised, the patient is at the mercy of staff attentiveness in maintaining continence. Too often, after waiting patiently for assistance that is not forthcoming, the patient simply must wet the bed.

There are several neurogenic and physiologic sources of fecal and urinary incontinence that may or may not be remediable. The source of any disorder must be thoroughly explored to determine cause, however. Even in organic disorders, training programs will usually minimize the frequency of accidents, which can be a great saving in both time and expense. However, when no organic causes of incontinence can be determined, then one must look for psychologic needs that may be met by the behavior. According to Ouslander (1981), incontinence may also be an oblique bid for attention or an expression of hostility or anger.

Inappropriate voiding can be due to confusion, drugged sleep, disorientation to the bathroom, or a purposeful effort to get attention or express anger. The behavior results in large amounts of staff time involved in unpleasant tasks, increased linen bills, low employee morale, hazardous conditions on the ward, catheterization, and a pervasive smell of urine in the facility.

When the cause of inappropriate voiding is to get staff attention, it often involves the need for tactile stimulation as well as verbal interaction. Obviously, there are appropriate ways to fill these needs that must be routinely provided if the incontinence is to be relinquished. In addition, the staff should be instructed to interact with the individual following this behavior in a straightforward manner, showing neither disgust nor condescension. The patient should be required to clean the area of urine and change clothing immediately.

If an individual urinates in an inappropriate receptacle, it may be for convenience or lack of motivation to go to the bathroom. This is often accompanied by other signs of poor motivation, such as poor grooming, inattention to personal hygiene, and low activity levels. Motivation may be increased by concerted attention by staff to grooming the individual and consistently encouraging and praising any efforts toward self-care. A commode or urinal may be made readily accessible.

In progressive dementia, a patient may have insufficient stimulus control. Urination is often preceded by precursor responses, such as exposure of the genitals, as the individual seeks to meet his or her need to void. Urination may occur in objects that seem like a toilet, such as a chair or a basin. In these cases, a bright colored symbol can be painted on the restroom door, the toilet seat may be painted the same bright color, and the individual conditioned to look for that stimulus when feeling the need to void. Lights are available that are activated by motion and these could be installed near the door to the toilet to stimulate interest and provide good lighting to encourage voiding in the appropriate place.

Programs to combat incontinence in long-term care settings are usually quite successful but require patience and persistence on the part of staff as well as patients. Such obvious things as night lights, access to toilets, and limitation of fluids just prior to bedtime are helpful. It is also essential to time the dispensation of diuretics in the early morning to avoid the need to get up during the night. All of these actions are easily implemented and logical, yet in some settings they are not given due attention.

EATING DISORDERS

Nutrition in older adults is often a problem. Feeding problems in severely demented patients include:

Lack of interest in food.
Inability to concentrate on eating.
Interference of primitive reflexes.
Disturbing tongue movements.
Hoarding of food in mouth.
Leakage of food from mouth.
Dysphagia.

Specific strategies must be identified and staff educated in methods to enhance the experience of eating. Several studies have shown various degrees of malnutrition to be common in the impaired elderly. Some of these are unquestionably due to the difficulties experienced in feeding. Eating disorders, such as bulimia, anorexia, and rumination, have been viewed as diseases of the young but recently more elders have been identified that are afflicted with an eating disorder. Larocca (1987) found that intergenerational support groups of those with eating disorders were effective in symptom resolution.

Anorexia in late life is quite common due to somatic problems, psychiatric conditions, medication regimens, and loss of interest in food. The energy requirements to maintain weight are reduced by about 30% so the selection of nutritious food in the required caloric intake is of more importance. Specific factors that tend to give rise to malnutrition are low levels of physical activity, drugs that alter the taste of foods, nonconducive meal environment, poor oral status and dentition, insufficient knowledge of nutrients, and unsuitable distribution of meals throughout the day.

Nutritional problems may relate to apathy, depression, need for attention, dementias, paranoia, food idiosyncrasies, cultural preferences, energy deficits, subliminal suicidal intent, dysphagias, and disinterest. Clearly, the remedy will be closely related to the cause.

Behavioral Influence of Foods

Kolata (1982) reports that, though the effects are subtle, numbers of studies confirm that certain foods affect behavior in predictable ways. Numerous articles have alerted the laity that red dye, sugar, and some additives may stimulate hyperactivity in children. Though some of those conclusions are suspect and even scientifically discounted, caregivers still must ask what effects will certain nutrients have on the behavior of frail elders, whom they know are more reactive to many substances than young adults. In effect, do caregivers "feed" their problems?

In this regard, tryptophan and its relationship to the production of serotonin has received the most attention by researchers regarding its soporific qualities. Serotonin is a neurotransmitter that is synthesized in the brain and that influences sleep, eating, locomotor activity, aggression, and pain sensitivity. In contrast to the assumption that a high protein meal would provide the tryptophan necessary for serotonin synthesis, it has been found that a high carbohydrate meal facilitates insulin release and the uptake of amino acids. Thus, a high carbohydrate meal and 1 gm of tryptophan were more effective in producing restful sleep than a high protein meal. There also seems to be a significant reduction in pain perception with high levels of brain serotonin.

Tyrosine is an amino acid that is precursor to dopamine and norepinephrine, which play a role in regulating motor activity and mood. A deficiency in catecholamines is supposed to make elders more subject to depression. Some studies reported by Kolata (1982) indicate that tyrosine intake was useful in relieving depression.

There is much yet to be done in research on the influence of diet on the biochemistry of the brain. Long-term care institutions provide an ideal setting for investigative studies of the effects of dietary changes on the behavior of the aged. As a beginning, it may be useful to observe, monitor, and change the dietary intake of individuals who are depressed, aggressive, or insomniac.

Dentition

Dentition is often neglected as a potential cause of poor eating habits. If problems in chewing are suspected, pureed foods may be given without further efforts to remedy the difficulty. Assessment of dentition could be a routine aspect of admission to long-term care programs. Some dentists and dental schools provide service to patients who need such attention.

For example, Catherine had lived in a nursing home for 12 years and managed to eat well in spite of having only three teeth that didn't match. She refused pureed foods and enjoyed the daily challenge of chopping her food into small bits. It gave her something to do and also the feeling of being involved in the preparation of her food, but Catherine was unique. Many residents simply abandon the effort to eat if dentition is poor or dental plates fit improperly.

Environment

The effects of dining room environment and food service procedures on demented patients may also be significant. The dining room should have few distractions. This is much easier said than done but for demented patients who are easily distracted from eating it may be useful to have a separate, small dining area with sound-absorbing draperies and dull tile floors rather than those that are bright and polished. Ideally, two persons would sit at a table and only four to a room. Given the dearth of such rooms in some facilities, it might be possible to use a patient's room and bring in two card tables. In addition, only one food should be served at a time. Demented patients tend to become absorbed in mixing and playing with food when there are more. When these procedures were followed for four to six weeks, the patients were returned to the large dining room but they continued to be given only one food at a time. This study, conducted in the geropsychiatric unit of the Veterans Administration Medical Center at Salisbury, North Carolina in 1984, demonstrated improved dietary intake and less playing with food among the four participants.

Dysphagia

Cuizon-Saiz (1988), in a personal communication, addressed the management of a dysphagic patient's nutritional needs. A 60-year-old male Caucasian patient with residual stroke damage that affected his left side and his speech had great difficulty swallowing. The staff found that if he was sitting in an upright position with a pillow bolstering his left side he could swallow with more ease. The emotional significance and life satisfaction of eating are not to be ignored. It is worth taking time and special effort to assist the dysphagic to eat rather than resort too quickly to artificial feeding. Dysphagics are generally able to swallow if the following principles are observed:

Maintain a relaxed and unhurried atmosphere.

Address the individual's fear of choking and provide reassurance that special techniques will reduce that problem.

Position the individual as nearly straight upright as possible.

Provide foods that have a semismooth and formed consistency (the consistency of stiffly whipped potatoes).

Ground or finely chopped foods are easier to swallow than those that are pureed.

Dry foods must be moistened enough to provide lubrication for ease of swallowing.

Fluids are best managed through a straw.

Pause for rest between each bite and remind the individual to swallow after each bite.

Although all staff in health care facilities should be trained in the Heimlich maneuver, it is particularly important that no staff feed a dysphagic client without prior demonstration of the mastery of this skill.

> Nutrition for the dysphagic patient can be a real nursing challenge. For the client, it is discouraging and can be frightening. Maintaining the ability of the individual to feed him or herself is basic to self-esteem. Power (1986) has given the following suggestions to enhance success:
>
> Multisensorial pleasant impact and moderate serving temperatures are of great value.
>
> Small bits of food that tend to choke patient or get lost in mouth should be combined with other foods to form a bolus. In other words, give peas with mashed potatoes, not separately.

Foods that crumble, such as dry toast, cookies, crackers, and cheddar cheese, should be avoided.

Food that is sticky or of thick consistency exhausts the client; avoid peanut butter, caramel, etc.

Clients with excess mucus production should avoid citrus juices, concentrated sweets, and milk products.

Consistent consumption of certain foods of client preference gives a sense of security. Variety in nutrients is needed but changes in foods must meet client approval.

Direct observation at mealtime is essential to ensure client mastery.

Frozen liquids are useful to strengthen muscles through sucking and are easier to manage without choking, for many clients.

Adapted from Power, Shirley (1986). "A Nutritional Challenge: The Elderly Patient with Dysphagia" by S. Power, 1986, *Gerontion* 1(2):12–13.

Suspiciousness

The elderly person who is extremely suspicious or paranoid may refuse to eat due to fear of poisoning. This is a phenomenon less common among elders than younger persons but it must be considered a possibility. This can be assessed by observing the patient's attempts to ignore his or her own food but take that of others (this is a common problem among demented patients and not indicative in those cases). The individual may also be seen smelling or carefully examining food given to him or her. These patients will often select most of the food they consume from snack trays, juice carts, fruit bowls, or other places in which general access to food is expected but individuals have a choice. Due to the chronic low level nature of paranoia in the old, it is best to adapt to the patient's needs and allow more frequent access to food sources that allow patient selection. The basic dynamic of the behavior is anxiety and feelings of powerlessness. Providing choices, reducing demands, and making the environment as predictable and secure as possible will approach the root of the problem and suspiciousness should diminish.

Hoarding Food

Hidden food may be a real issue in the control of rodents and insects. No information could be found in the literature that addresses this problem but some facility staff have found solutions to this rather common occurrence. One nursing assistant recognized the cohort effects of the depression years and the tendency toward hoarding that grew out of the deprivation. She initiated discussion with the patient about her experience during that time and found that she had been hungry many times. Thereafter, she made certain the patient had some individually packaged crackers in her room at all times. Sometimes hoarding may be symptomatic of generalized insecurity or territorial needs. Each person must have a place that is sacrosanct and not invaded by others. When this is not provided, caregivers can expect troublesome behaviors.

Personal Preferences

Food idiosyncrasies may be due to unusual habits of eating, poor judgment, or, as in the following example (Cuizon-Saiz, 1988), a family's attempts to cope with the difficult problems of an aged member.

> A 79-year-old woman with advanced Alzheimer's disease and chronic pulmonary obstructive disease refused to eat upon admission to a nursing home. She pushed and verbally abused the caregivers who attempted to feed her. A staff conference was called to consider ways to induce her to eat. Several considerations were discussed: was this an adjustment reaction to anger over her institutionalization; was she frightened of the individuals she did not recognize; was her dentition adequate for comfortable chewing; was she intent on suicide; had she an extreme energy deficit; or had she simply lost interest in food? As nutritional habits are sometimes not discussed during the admission process and recognizing that her past nutritional history was important the director of nursing contacted the family. They informed her that the effort of chewing and eating often increased Mrs. B.'s shortness of breath and that she had been subsisting on a liquid diet for some time. With this information, staff kept high protein supplements of various flavors at her bedside. In order to attract her attention, they were placed on a bright colored placemat. Given the availability and freedom to drink them as she desired, she consumed four to six each day. Though she was taken to the dining room for each meal, she frequently ate nothing or only a few bites; however, her weight was maintained by the supplements. As the staff felt less need to urge her to eat, she did not display hostility and began to eat a little more.

Cultural and personal preferences in food may go unmet in settings where the meal planning is not done in the facility. One administrator of a nursing home in San Francisco said food purchases and dietary plans are carried out in the corporate offices and the individual facility has little opportunity to alter it. In such cases, it may be possible to engage family members in bringing desired foods to the patient. It would also be important for administrative staff to advocate for more flexibility in meal planning. The routine choice of dietary staples, such as rice, potatoes, or beans is not expensive and may markedly add to the satisfaction and nutritional intake of some residents. Patient council meetings are often focused on complaints about food. While it is recognized that these complaints may be an expression of general dissatisfaction, it is yet important to respond to expressed wishes of clients and life-long habits. A creative response to personal preference can include encouraging residents to submit their favorite recipes to the cook who would prepare them.

Depressed and apathetic elders simply ignore food. Anorexia may become entrenched as the problem is compounded. The less they eat, the less they desire to eat. Energy and interest in life is further diminished by the nutritional deficits. Wichita (1977) established a reminiscing group at mealtime for several depressed and apathetic elders who had lost interest in eating. The membership of the group was consistent and a nursing assistant ate with the group at each meal. As she initiated discussions of foods the group members had enjoyed earlier, they became more interested in eating. Other memories of a pleasant nature were also discussed. The group became more social and animated as they continued to meet together and the benefits of mealtime reminiscing were more extensive than had been anticipated. See Chapter 4 for additional information on reminiscence groups.

Ethics of Feeding

In regard to nasogastric tube feeding for elders who refuse to eat, ethical issues have been given extensive attention. It is thought that many elders refuse to eat in an attempt at starvation though they may not overtly admit it. Nonetheless, caregivers are put in a difficult position if the competency of the individual is in question. Each state has different regulations in regard to whether allowing an individual to starve may be considered passive euthanasia and thus have legal implications. The caregiver must consider these carefully. In addition, there are symbolic and emotional meanings of food that may urge caregivers to force feed in the name of comfort and basic care. When at all possible, however, allow the individual the right to refuse food. That may be the only means available of expressing autonomy and dignity in dying.

Callahan (1985), a notable ethicist, discusses the feeding of the dying elderly and whether withholding food can be considered neglect or abuse. Is it morally acceptable to withhold food in the case of the severely demented or comatose elderly? There are arguments pro and con. One must consider whether artificial food and hydration are medical treatments or basic requirements of care; what policies and restrictions are necessary to guide decisions and ensure consistency; or should the decision be individual, based on knowledge of the life patterns and supposed intent of the person no longer able to make a decision? Long held traditions of medical care support the idea that it is a general moral duty to feed the hungry and give water to those who thirst. Caregivers must also be aware that lurking deep within them is a propensity to neglect the powerless, the burdensome, and the inconvenient. Because withholding food and water can lead to a coarsening of human sensibilities toward the dying and critically ill, Callahan was hesitant to do so. The natural repugnance against such actions would need to be individually overcome and, in the process, could dull compassion. Should caregivers allow fears about abuses to overshadow the possible benefits to old people who no longer have the capacity to participate as members of the human community? Caregivers are moving into an era when the increasing human and economic burden of prolonging life is a persistent issue. While caregivers do not yet have answers, they must attempt to cautiously make humane and wise decisions.

CONCLUSION

In this chapter, I have addressed the major and common behavioral problems that occur in a small percentage of the aged population. When concentrating on these problems, which are seen frequently in institutional settings, caregivers must remember that the vast majority of the aged function very well and cope effectively with social roles and expectations, and find satisfaction in life.

6

Psychogeriatric Disorders: Causes and Care

This chapter focuses on psychogeriatric disorders that predominate in late life. Functional psychiatric disorders are rooted in losses, uncertainty, and previous disorders that persist into old age. Often, they do not come to the attention of mental health professionals until the effects are disabling. Organic psychiatric disorders, often of mixed origin, are prevalent among elders who are hospitalized. Behavioral problems discussed in the previous chapter provide observable evidence of psychologic and emotional disorders that have been expressed in an oblique manner. This chapter, then, will explore the nature of the underlying disorders that have exacerbated and command immediate attention by mental health professionals. In addition, because of their disabling effects, such disorders will usually precipitate hospitalization in a mental health unit. These disorders are defined by the Diagnostic Statistical Manual III R and will be presented in those categories.

DIAGNOSES OF THE PSYCHOGERIATRIC CLIENT

In planning appropriate care for the mentally disturbed elder, one must discriminate between a life-long pattern of mental and emotional problems versus the onset of mental disorders in late life. Life-long problems are likely to exacerbate in old age due to weakening of defensive mechanisms related to general reduction in coping energies physically or psychically. As one ages, some earlier mental disorders are likely to become more pronounced. When problems occur in clinically observable form for the first time in later life, it may also be due to loss of adaptational energy or lack of incentive. In some elders, it is delightful to see them for the first time demonstrating a reduction of inhibition and less concern with social and cultural inhibitions. In other older persons, the loss of inhibitions may go beyond tolerable bounds. Since so much of what is considered mentally aberrant is bound to cultural and social expectations, caregivers must be reluctant to label any behavior as pathologic if it serves the individual's adaptation and does not hinder others. These cautionary words are precedent to attempting to encourage clarity in diagnosis and care planning. Of all persons, the aged are most likely to be misdiagnosed. For example, Organic Brain Syndrome (OBS) was for years a wastebasket diagnosis. In other words, those persons with such a diagnosis were deemed incurable, and almost literally thrown away. Now, we must guard against the indiscriminate use of the diagnosis of Alzheimer's disease. Alert caregivers will continually provide additional data to confirm, refine, or challenge intake diagnoses. In this regard, data suggest that a high incidence of paranoid symptoms are classified under the rubric of atypical disorders, thus paranoid disorder subtypes need to be clarified; manic episodes persist into old age as evidenced by geropsychiatric populations studied; schizophrenic disorders are infrequently initially diagnosed in late life due to age and time restrictions in the criteria.

In old age, the most frequent categorically diagnosable psychiatric problems fall in the category of Adjustment Disorders, followed closely by Mood Disorders, Sleep Disorders, Somatoform Disorders, and Organic Mental Disorders. Nor are these necessarily mutually exclusive. For instance, when one has a mood disorder, he or she will likely have sleep disorders and somatoform disorders as well. For purposes of management, it is necessary to define the most blatant or troublesome problem as if it were discrete in order to apply orderly logic to its solution. To assist in doing so, I have identified the most likely mental problems of the aged that might reasonably be expected to relate to the psychiatric diagnosis (see Appendices and Table 6.1). The life-saving and prolonging focus of most acute-care interventions possible in our present health care system make it imperative that caregivers rapidly and properly identify clients' needs. Appropriate care plans cannot be limited to the brief hospitalizations that are now common but must include comprehensive discharge plans.

TABLE 6.1   Etiology of Categorical Mental Disorders

Organic mental disorders and syndromes:
  Reduced homeostatic resilience results in confusion and incapacitation in situations of deteriorating health
  Disturbance in self-concept occurs with inability to incorporate environmental feedback
  Chronic disease processes reduce coping energies
  Compromised organ function produces adverse reactions to drugs
Sleep and arousal disorders:
  Sleep patterns are more easily disrupted after age 60
  Daytime activity reduction results in poor sleep patterns
  Hypoxia interrupts progressive stages of sleep
  Deep, restful (stage 4) sleep is not attained in late life
  Individuals are more responsive to environmental stimuli as a result of not attaining deep sleep levels
Delusional disorders:
  Isolated lifestyles reduce interactional corrective feedback when thought processes become skewed
  Victimization occurs more frequently when one is old and feels helpless
  Ageist attitudes are internalized by the frail old
Mood disorders:
  Neurotransmitter production is reduced in old age and individuals are more prone to depression
  Significant losses occur with more frequency in late life
  Physical deterioration erodes trust and optimism
  Awareness of impending death may create despair
Anxiety disorders:
  Predictability is eroded for reasons above
  Maintaining rituals and compulsive behaviors may require too much energy
Somatoform disorders:
  Realities of chronic illness and functional limitations predispose one to expectation of further health problems
  Hypochondriasis is an overt expression of depression
Gender and sexual disorders:
  Illness and lowered energy reduces libido
  Overindulgence in food and alcohol creates temporary impotence
  Ageist myths about asexuality in late life may be internalized
  Vascular problems create impotence in men
Adjustment disorders:
  Requirements for major readjustments in lifestyle and self-concept occur in situations of functional limitations due to chronic illness, enforced retirement, relocation, decreased mobility, reduced income, and changes in family relationships.
Personality disorders:
  May become more pronounced due to weakening of defense mechanisms or less concern about monitoring behaviors or maintaining social facades
Issues to consider, not attributable to a mental disorder:
  Borderline intellectual functioning related to lack of opportunity for formal education (more likely in the very old)
  Antisocial behavior, such as shoplifting, related to need

TABLE 6.1 (continued)

Uncomplicated bereavement related to real loss and experienced as severe depression resolved in time
Noncompliance with medical treatment related to inadequate understanding or subliminal suicide intent
Phase of life problems related to real issues of personal mortality, meaninglessness, and reduced capacities
Marital problems related to long-standing problems or aging at different rates
Parent–child problems related to changing roles and expectations as parents become dependent

Because DRGs do not presently place prospective reimbursement caps on frank psychiatric diagnoses, geropsychiatric care settings are in a somewhat better position than the medical counterparts. However, most often the mental health problems of the aged are intermingled with physical problems and the diagnosis is much more likely to have an organic/somatic base than a functional psychiatric label. The organic/functional discrimination of psychiatric nomenclature is separate from functional assessment of the capacity to perform activities of daily living. In psychiatry, functional simply means there is no measureable systemic or organic change that can account for the symptoms the individual is displaying. In geriatrics, functional is related to an individual's capacity for self-care and the activities of daily living. It is indeed a significant issue in terms of relative dependence/independence.

ORGANIC MENTAL DISORDERS AND SYNDROMES

One of the greatest challenges to health professionals is to accurately differentiate among dementias, deliriums, and depressions. This type of diagnostic activity is theoretically limited to physicians and gerontologic nurse practitioners. In reality, because of the nature and subtlety of symptoms, the attending nurses are likely to have more behavioral data on which to make a diagnostic judgment than those caregivers who have less exposure to the patient. The characteristics, onset, progression, duration, behavioral features, and accompanying emotions all are factors that must be considered in arriving at an appropriate delineation of the problem. Table 6.2 is useful in recognizing differences in the disorders. It is extremely important these discriminations be made. Incorrectly diagnosed and treated, disorders that are potentially reversible become irreversible dementias. Though each disorder has specific characteristics, they may be difficult to discern—all three conditions may

TABLE 6.2   Characteristics of Dementia, Delirium and Depression

Dementia	Delirium	Depression
Symptoms:		
Loss of intellect	Clouded consciousness	Anhedonia
Memory loss	Perceptual disturbance	Mood changes
mild-forgetful	Disordered thoughts	Memory loss
moderate	Disorientation	Somatic complaints
severe	Memory impairment	/hypochondriasis
Attention	Fluctuating moods	Apathy
easily distracted		Flat affect
		Rumination
		Indecision
Onset:		
Variable	Short, rapid, abrupt	Usually clearly related
depending on cause		to recent events
Duration:		
May be reversible or	Reversible	Treatable-lifting in 3 to
irreversible	Usually one week to one	6 months
Up to 12 years	month	May be chronic
		Suicide rate high
Behavior:		
Sleep pattern reversed	Sleep/wakefulness	Sleep impaired
Symptoms worse at	impaired	Slowing/retarded
night	Fluctuations in mood and	movement
Incontinence	actions	Withdrawal
Trouble learning new	Tremor	Agitation
tasks	Speech incoherent or	Poor coordination
Impaired judgment	limited	Aware of deficits
Poor impulse control		
Language difficulties		
Personality change		
Emotions:		
Early stages anxiety and	Disturbed	Distressed
depression	Variable	Disturbed
Vulnerability	Labile	Guilt
Delusional	Fear/panic	Low self-esteem
Suspicious	Euphoria	Hopelessness
		Helplessness

Adapted from J. Gallo, W. Reichel & L. Andersen. (1988). *Handbook of geriatric assessment.* Rockville, MD: Aspen.

K. Ronsman. (1988). Pseudodementia. *Geriatric Nursing, 9,* 50–52.

J. Dreyfus. (1988). Depression assessment and interventions in the medically ill elderly. *Journal of Gerontological Nursing, 14,* 27–35.

exist simultaneously in one individual. For example, a person in the early stages of an organic mental disorder will most certainly be depressed at the realization of waning mental capacities; in addition, due to the compromised cerebral function, any infection, systemic deficits, injuries, or substance exposure will produce concurrent delirium.

SUBSTANCE-INDUCED MENTAL DISORDERS

Substance-induced mental disorders are more frequent in the aged than in younger populations and should be the first line of investigation when cognitive impairment is noted. This does not indicate that older persons are more prone than younger persons to substance abuse but that they are much more likely to have adverse reactions to substances. Reduced homeostatic resilience, compromised organ function, presence of chronic disease processes, and the likelihood of reliance on several prescription drugs in the management of various conditions all predispose the elder person to substance-induced mental confusion of a temporary nature (see the discussion on pharmacology in Chapter 4).

Expressions of impaired mental function, whatever the etiology, are likely to result in catastrophic reactions and uncharacteristic explosive outbursts. These reactions must be interpreted as indicative of panic states and a decompensation of coping capacities. Nursing actions then must be directed toward restoring a sense of security and control within the capacities of the frightened and impaired individual.

SLEEP AND AROUSAL DISORDERS

Sleep and arousal disorders of late life are usually secondary to disease processes, are substance induced, or are normal sleep patterns that seem abnormal to the individual. It is most important to ensure the individual that daytime napping is not detrimental to night sleep and is, in fact, expected to increase in healthy old age. In addition, it is useful to educate the elder to expected changes in sleep patterns: during the decade of the 60s there is a noticeable decrease in the depth of sleep and more frequent wakenings during the night. Because stage 4 level of sleep is never attained, one may waken feeling less refreshed. Sleep patterns of males also change earlier than those of females. Both are likely to experience changes before age 70, however. Sleep patterns in those who are demented are grossly disorganized and become a most troubling symptom for families and caregivers to manage. Tolerating night wandering becomes a significant issue. In this respect, the nurse can assist

174   Caring for the Psychogeriatric Client

the family to think of ways to make the environment safe to the greatest extent possible. A simple hook latch placed far above eye level on the door leading downstairs is a creative and effective way of safety-proofing the environment. Unfortunately, it is not usually effective to try and modify the schedule to induce sleep at a more reasonable time. It is always helpful to make the environment peaceful, reduce stimuli, and keep soft lights burning to dispel anxiety. Music with soft rhythm and a cadence in synchrony with heart beat has been found soothing by some music therapists. See discussion of disturbed sleep in Chapter 5.

DELUSIONAL DISORDERS

Persecutory delusions are often evidence of internalized ageist messages of social origins as well as those that are self-imposed. Undoubtedly, this is the most notable evidence of the ultimate impact of societal feedback and perceived rejection. Certainly, it lends credence to the symbolic interactionist concept of human adaptation. In some individuals, it is possible to trace, over time, the gradual fulmination of a sense of victimization that ultimately becomes a full-fledged, intricate paranoid delusion. Caution must be observed in arriving at this diagnosis; however, lack of caution can prove disastrous. For example, it is common for those intimately involved with the elderly to have seen the abuse, persecution, deprivation, fraud, and chicanery inflicted on an unsuspecting individual simply because of misdiagnosis. The stories are sometimes quite unbelievable, especially when involving those of betrayal by spouse or children. Sorting fact from fiction may be difficult. As with all delusional systems, when anxiety is reduced, the need for the delusion is also reduced. Therefore, it is necessary to carefully attend to individual process as well as content of the thoughts expressed.

MOOD DISORDERS

Depressive disorders are so common in late life some gerontologists believe that successful aging is largely dependent on an individual's capacity for coping with depressive episodes. Of course, there are reasons why the aged become depressed more frequently: natural mood altering cerebral substances are less effectively secreted in the later years; situations that involve loss occur with more frequency; physical and psychic coping energies are gradually depleted in normal aging processes; illness, when it occurs, always has some depressive components; disappointment with one's life and the sure knowledge that little time is left may give a sense of futility; and anticipatory grief related to one's own demise can be personally devastating.

ANXIETY DISORDERS

By far the most common evidence of anxiety states among old people will be obsessive compulsive disorders. The more threatened they feel, the tighter they will cling to ritualized behaviors that provide a sense of order in perceived chaos. Jarvik and Russell (1979) identified and described another way anxiety is expressed as a state of "vigilant watchfulness" in which the individual may give the impression of being withdrawn or apathetic. On closer observation, it is noted that the person is in a semicatatonic state. This response to intense anxiety was labeled the "freeze" reaction and thought to occur particularly among the frail old who lack the energy to fight or flee a perceived threat.

SOMATOFORM DISORDERS

It is unclear how often somatization is a primary response to unmet psychological needs or unidentified conflicts. Unfortunately, the literature does not address this in relation to an aged population. Due to the fact that 80% of the aged have at least one chronic health problem and over half experience some functional limitations related to chronic illness, it would be difficult to delineate purely somatoform disorders. Even the hypochondriasis so familiar to nurses who work with the depressed elderly may be rooted in an awareness of general physical deterioration as well as a response to a mood disorder. A general caution here is to assume there is a legitimate physical problem until shown otherwise. Do insist the older person do everything possible for him or herself and avoid any action that will increase dependency. This is at no time as important as in late life when the adage "use it or lose it" is particularly true related to individual function and management of activities of daily living (ADLs).

GENDER AND SEXUAL DISORDERS

Males who are healthy continue to function sexually into very late years if they desire to do so. Some even father children in their 70s and beyond. Their sexual patterns, though with naturally diminished penile turgidity, frequency of intercourse, and delayed ejaculation, remain much as in their youth. If the individual was highly active in youth, he will tend to remain more active in late life than others who were less interested in sexual activity.

The most troublesome problem is inability to achieve erection. This may be due to overindulgence in food and alcohol, debilitation, disease processes (particularly diabetes or vascular insufficiency), psychological reactions of boredom with the sexual partner, or internalized ageist myths.

Fortunately, in recent years advances have been made in combating both physical and psychological barriers to satisfying intercourse. Penile implants are now available that are effective and aesthetically acceptable. Papaverine will create a temporary erection when injected at the base of the penis. Other drugs are being used experimentally that seem to have aphrodisiac qualities. There are numbers of urologists who specialize in dealing with sexual problems of a mechanical origin. Psychological issues are best approached by couples in order to maximize mutually acceptable resolutions. There are now sex counselors in most communities. Resource information may be obtained from the Sex Information and Education Council of the United States (SIECUS) (see appendices).

Women have quite different sexual issues to deal with in old age. In spite of increasing friability of vaginal tissue, diminished lubrication, and shrinkage of the vaginal vault, many women retain a strong sexual desire in late life. The greatest problem in expressing sexuality through intercourse is the lack of available and capable partners, however. Other mechanical problems are often due to arthritic changes that may make certain coital positions uncomfortable. Of course, this can be remedied by the use of other positions or sexual expressions.

Orgasmic disorders of older women are probably quite common though studies have not been found that focus on age differences in this respect. Vibrators will produce orgasm in women who have the physical response capacity; however, they may find them unacceptable. It is incumbent on nurses working with the aged to be sensitive to their generational differences and expectations. Given the opportunity to discuss sexuality and intimacy, some elders may remain reticent and this must be respected.

ADJUSTMENT DISORDERS

Adjustment disorders are seen as reactions to developmental or environmental stressors that occur within three months of the onset of the event. The most commonly observed of these among the aged population are: chronic illness with functional limitations, enforced retire-ment, undesired relocation, abrupt reduction of income, diminished involvement in community due to loss of driver's license, and deterio-ration in family relationships due to unanticipated needs and de-mands.

Adjustment disorders of aging with any or all of the predominant moods and behaviors will be primarily observed by nurses in the community. Those nurses in institutions will be aware of them as secondary to the admitting diagnoses. Most of the persons demon-strating such disorders do not come to the attention of health care personnel until the natural caregivers (spouse, family) are depleted.

PERSONALITY DISORDERS

Personality disorders may be more pronounced in old age than in youth, only because all personality traits tend to become stronger and more visible in the process of aging. Neugarten (1968) noted that elders become, in a sense, caricatures of their younger selves. This may be due to a weakening of the defenses that monitor personality or it may be purely because older persons are less likely to exert energy in maintaining facades.

Personality disorders are inflexible traits that inhibit individual growth and personal development. They include categories of para-noia, dependency, obsessive/compulsive, and passive/aggressive types. Paranoia as a personality disorder is inhibiting and rooted in a basic lack of trust. It is dealt with later in the chapter. Dependency develops in proportion to the thwarting of initiative and becomes an element of personality when opportunities for self-care are consis-tently denied. It is most often accompanied by depression and has been discussed under that category. Excessive reliance on ritual and order can become disabling if it overrides spontaneous expression of feelings. It is thought that obsessional and compulsive personalities are compensating for unruly aspects of self to provide security against losing control. The passive/aggressive personality is bound in fear of losing the love he so desperately needs if he is not quietly compliant. Often he finds subversive ways to get his unique needs met. Underly-ing all of these is a persistent disturbance in self-concept. That was discussed quite thoroughly in Chapter 2.

The more obscure personality disorders such as the borderline, the histrionic, the narcissistic, the antisocial, and the schizoid can be found in young and old but the grating aspects of these personalities are often tempered by life experience and maturity even though in some they fulminate to uncomfortable proportions. The most important thing to remember is that personality traits have been adaptive to the individual's survival and will be modified only to the extent that needs can be met more directly and reliably.

ORGANIC CAUSES OF PSYCHOLOGIC DISORDERS

It is well known that any interference with cerebral perfusion, hypoxia, drug reactions, endocrine dysfunctions, and any disease of the central nervous system will result in psychologic disorders of an organic source. Less often recognized but just as frequent are psychologic reactions to urinary tract infections or upper respiratory infections. These are usually seen as minor problems and often the ramifications in terms of confusion or behavioral responses is overlooked.

Persons with organic dementia exhibit many problem behaviors but there is a remarkable lack of consistency in relation to disease process or progress. Why do some demonstrate delusions, others anxiety or agitation, and yet others depression or hallucinations? As these reactions occur in only a fraction of individuals with dementia, it behooves caregivers to show caution in categorizing them as the inevitable symptoms accompanying progressive dementia.

The aged have a small margin between compensated levels of hypoxemia and intolerable hypoxia. This is due primarily to vascular bed changes and a relatively fixed cardiac output. Early symptoms are often seen as delirium, paranoia, or agitation. Given this knowledge, any condition or medication that decreases cerebral profusion may be seen as undesirable. As a result the sometimes indiscriminate use of diuretics must be addressed more frequently. The old adage of adding 10 points to diastolic blood pressure for each decade after age 70 may have some wisdom behind it (Kane, Ouslander, & Abrass, 1989).

MEDICAL DISORDERS AND PSYCHIATRIC SYMPTOMS

Schaffer and Donlon (1983) have identified certain medical disorders that often present as psychiatric symptoms in the elderly. Often they are the only clinical evidence of an underlying physical illness. To avoid permanent organic brain damage, these disorders must be detected and reversed as quickly as possible. Table 6.3 lists the major psychiatric disorders and the potential physical illnesses that should be ruled out. These are particularly important when the referral for mental health services has come from a social agency or a source that

TABLE 6.3   Common Medical Causes of Psychiatric Symptoms

Depression
  Medications
    Antihypertensives
    Corticosteroids
    L-dopa
    CNS depressants
  Infections
    Hepatitis
    Chronic pyelonephritis
    Subacute bacterial endocarditis
  Endocrine
    Hypothyroidism
    Diabetes
    Addison's disease
  Neoplasms
    Brain
    Lung
  Neurologic
    Dementia
    Parkinson's disease
  Miscellaneous
    Uremia
    Anemia
    Dehydration
Mania
  Medications
    Corticosteroids
    Isoniazid
    Procarbazine
    Amphetamines
  Metabolic
    Postoperative recovery
    Hemodialysis
  Infection
    Influenza
    CNS syphilis
  Neoplasm
    Metastatic squamous adenocarcinoma
    Certain rare brain tumors
Schizophreniform pyschosis
  Medications (toxic levels)
    Sympathomimetics
    Anti-inflammatory agents
    Tricyclics and MAD antidepressants
    Anticholinergics

(continued)

TABLE 6.3   (continued)

Central nervous system disorders
   Temporal lobe disorders
   Multiple sclerosis
   Systemic lupus erythematosis
   Neoplasms
   CNS syphilis
   Endocrine disorders
      Hyper and hypothyroidism
      Addison's disease
   Miscellaneous
      Alcoholic hallucinations
      Pernicious anemia
      Deafness
Delirium
   Medications
      Antidepressants
      Antipsychotics
      Lithium
      Anticholinergics
      CNS depressants
   Infections
      Pneumonia
      Urinary tract infections
      Sepsis
   Metabolic
      Hypoxia
      Renal failure (azotemia)
      Hepatic failure
      Electrolyte imbalance
   Endocrine
      Hyper and hypothyroidism
      Diabetes
   Cardiovascular
      Myocardial infarct
      Cardiac arrhythmias
      Congestive heart failure
   Miscellaneous
      Fecal impaction
      Dehydration
      Bladder distention
      Anemia
      Environmental change, particularly at night
Dementia
   Neurological
      Primary degenerative disease (Alzheimer's)
      Parkinson's disease

TABLE 6.3   (continued)

Infections
  Abcesses
  Encephalitis
  Meningitis
Medications
  Lithium toxicity
  Chronic alcoholism
  CNS depressants used over lengthy period
Metabolic/endocrine
  Hypoxia
  Hypoglycemia
  Pernicious anemia
Cerebrovascular
  CVA
  Cerebral atherosclerosis
Trauma
  Concussion
  Contusion
  Subdural hematoma
Neoplasms
  Primary brain tumor, advanced
  Extensive metasteses of cancer
Anxiety
Medications
  Withdrawal of CNS depressants
  Corticoteroids
  Xanthine derivatives
  Caffeine
Metabolic
  Hypoglycemia
  Hypoxia
Endocrine
  Hyperthyroidism
  Menopause
  Adrenal tumor
  Hyperparathyroidism
Neurological
  Early CNS degeneration
Cardiovascular
  Paroxysmal atrial tachycaria
  Prolapsed mitral valve

Reprinted from Schaffer, C. B.; Donlon, P. T. (1983).
Medical causes of psychiatric symptoms in the elderly.
Clinical Gerontologist 1983 1(4) 3–17.

has insufficient knowledge of etiologic issues. Suggestions for appropriate screening of elderly patients include:

- Recent changes in mental status should be considered a medical problem until proven otherwise.
- Medication and substance ingestion must be completely and carefully evaluated.
- Obtain a complete history of chronic or recurring medical disorders.
- Upon a first onset of major depression, psychosis, or mania a complete medical evaluation is essential.
- Visual hallucinations in the aged are most often organic in origin.
- Families and friends will be needed to obtain an accurate history of mental changes.
- Dementia and delirium can occur simultaneously in elderly patients.
- Any change in mental status should be evaluated aggressively as patients can deteriorate rapidly if there is an underlying medical disorder.

Medical problems that exacerbate or create psychologic problems are common in late life. It is estimated that 30 to 50% of hospitalized elderly experience some confusion and the majority of these cases go undetected. Increased mortality, longer hospital stay, and inappropriate transfers to nursing homes may result. The factors associated with the development of confusion have been largely speculative or derived from anecdotal accounts. As a result, there is a need for intensive investigation of the significance of cerebral metabolism, neural function, affective status, social dynamics, and environment in the contribution to confusion in the medically ill hospitalized elderly. The example below illustrates this point.

A student nurse spent the morning caring for an 80-year-old lady scheduled for gallbladder surgery. The woman was alert, lucid, and quite charming. She had rarely been hospitalized and considered herself to be in unusually good health for her age. Upon returning to care for this individual following her surgery, the student nurse was astonished to find her disoriented, delusional, and greatly agitated. The unit staff felt some of her medications may have induced these responses. However, the cause was never pursued or determined. The student nurse was able to be extremely helpful in assuring the woman that the confusion was a temporary reaction to the surgery and would soon subside. She remained with her and continuously gave corrective feedback and assisted her in accomplishing necessary activities. The most important intervention was the reassurance she provided. Later, the patient told her she had been worried that she had lost her reason and that it would never return.

Unfortunately, the most basic interventions, such as the one described in the example, are often neglected in the demands of giving technical nursing care. As a result, caregivers must constantly remind themselves of the patient's perspective and be available to assist the patient in understanding any bizarre or uncharacteristic reactions.

Wolanin and Phillips (1981) list several situations that are prodromal to confusion: hypothermia, dehydration, disruption in usual activities of daily living, and distortions in time and space cues. Body temperature regulating mechanisms may be disrupted due to medications and surgical procedures; dehydration is frequently a result of the various, and sometimes repeated, tests that require 12-hour fasting periods. In addition, elders may not be offered fluids frequently enough and may forget to ask for them. If one is on IV fluid replacement, it is still important to keep the client aware of the need for fluid. Disruption in usual activities of daily living is unavoidable when hospitalized. Caregivers may assist elders by encouraging them to carry on as much of their usual daily pattern as possible, and allowing them the time it takes to do things for themselves. Distortion in time and space cues is perhaps most blatant in acute hospitalization. Loudspeakers, lights, music, and activity round the clock mitigate against a clear perception of time markers when one is away from usual surroundings. Meals may be the only way one has to orient. Nurses can assess the need of the individual for cues and make an effort to modify the environment appropriately. For example, one mildly confused man in a psychiatric unit of a general hospital was further confused when his pillow case was stamped with the name of another hospital. How was he to know that the hospitals used a collective laundry and often received linens with the name of another hospital stamped boldly upon them.

Norris reports (1986) that the restlessness so often evident in hospitalized elders may be a result of disturbance in rhythmicity. To diagnose this possibility, one would assess the following:

Increased activity.
Repetitive activity.
Apparently purposeless activity.
Urgency of movements.
Increased muscle tone.

Though seemingly random and purposeless, this behavior is indicative of a transitional phase in which the organism is preparing to adapt to altered biorhythms. A similar effect has been noticed in some persons suffering jet-lag. It is useful for staff and patient to be aware that this is a transitional phase and to see it as process rather than as a constant.

Another aspect of the interplay of medical disorders and psychiatric symptoms was found by Haag and Stuhr (1987) in a systematic study of over 500 consecutive admissions to internal medicine wards. These investigators found a clear correspondence of 40% in the emergence of a disease process concurrent with emotionally relevant events, particularly those of loss. Even more significant was that only 5% of these elders were motivated to reflect on the significance. It was suggested that the elders may be oriented to the primary or secondary gain derived from physical disorders and unable to move beyond the somatic orientation.

In a critical review of literature related to the causes of dementia, Clarfield (1987) found 16% of all cases were potentially reversible. The most common causes of these reversible dementias were drugs, depression, and metabolic disorders. Kane, Ouslander, and Abrass (1989) have noted the apparent lack of attention to a relatively common disorder, hypothyroidism, and the mistaken diagnosis of dementia or depression that is often made.

Hypothyroidism in the elderly is, even when suspected, often incorrectly screened. T3 and T4 are inadequate measures to exclude hypothyroidism. Pomerantz and Meyer (1987) found that thyroid stimulating hormone (TSH) with or without thyrotropin releasing hormone (TRH) could correctly identify overt or "failing" thyroid syndrome. Cautious replacement therapy is advised. Initial and every six weeks incremental doses of L-thyroxine, 12.5 micrograms daily, were given as long as the TSH levels remained elevated. In no instance did any patient treated with this regimen manifest cardiovascular complications.

Patients with Parkinson's disease quite commonly develop insidious psychiatric changes after years of chronic therapy. However, because of its late emergence, the recognition of the source of the problem may be difficult. Psychiatric problems tend to emerge progressively, beginning with sleep disorders and progressing to nightmares and night terrors. As the disease progresses further, visual hallucinations, paranoia, and confusion may appear. Nurses must be aware of this potential in all patients with long-standing Parkinson's disease. In addition, nurses must alert the patient to this potentiality in order to reduce the anxiety and panic that may accompany such changes. It is important to remember that the extent of distress experienced by a Parkinsonian patient may not be adequately conveyed due to the bland facial expressions, lack of animation and affect that are characteristic of the disease.

Naughton (1987) reports the case of an older adult admitted to a geropsychiatric unit with a diagnosis of severe dementia. A thorough multidisciplinary evaluation established a diagnosis of depression and Parkinson's disease. This case serves to emphasize the need for more comprehensive assessments and the difficulty in arriving at appropriate diagnoses of persons with neurologic disorders that are accompanied by psychiatric symptoms.

DEMENTIAS

Dementias are probably the foremost concern of psychogeriatric clinicians. Often the therapeutic goals become lost or clouded in the awareness of long-term outcome. Since the progression of the disease process is relentless, it is difficult to maintain a focus on caring and quality of life. As a result, many facilities have care units for demented patients where caregivers make special efforts to provide quality of life.

Alzheimer's Disease

Alzheimer's disease is the most prevalent of the dementias and is characterized by the progressive and diffuse infiltration of functioning brain cells with neurofibrillary tangles and neuritic plaques. It is a disease process that, at present, has no known cause or cure despite extensive research during the last 15 years. Presently, the focus of research is on the discovery that acetylcholine is greatly reduced in the brain of Alzheimer's patients and on attempts to administer substances to compensate. Ingestion of Lethicin, the precursor to acetylcholine, has had disappointing results. Symptomatically, there is a steady loss of cognitive capacities, judgment, and ability to carry on the activities of daily living. The afflicted individual may survive from 2 to 15 years depending upon general physical status and the age at which the disease occurs. The younger the patient, the more virulent the disease. Most victims are cared for by their families until the burden of care becomes intolerable, at which time they are placed in a nursing home. The greatest current problem, however, is the tendency to assign a diagnosis of Alzheimer's disease too quickly and too frequently. Actual diagnosis can be ascertained only by microscopic examination of brain tissue. Therefore, caregivers must first assume that evidence of dementia may be reversible and every effort made to rule out causes other than Alzheimer's disease. When the diagnosis seems unmistakably evident, then the charge for caregivers is expressed by Mace and Rabins (1984, p. 44):

We can make a difference in whether such people suffer with their illness or whether they are comfortable and able to enjoy moment-to-moment. I believe our charge for the coming decade is to learn what we can do to rehabilitate patients, to enable them to live *with* their illness, to improve their function, to remove excess disability, and to improve their quality of life.

Ideally special care units should train all staff who interact with the Alzheimer's patient. Specific needs of the Alzheimer's patient include provision of a safe environment; companionship; understanding of nonverbal language; management of anxiety; dealing with reversed sleep patterns; provision of activities seven days a week; emphasis on ambulation; avoidance of reliance on drugs and restraints; and monitoring fluids, nutrition, and weight. When carefully planned and well managed, these units (or the training they provide to other caregivers) add appreciably to the quality of life of the Alzheimer's patients. Family support groups are also integral to unit function and patient management.

Most importantly, patients with Alzheimer's disease do remain responsive to the feeling tones of those around them. While they may not express warmth, satisfaction, or appreciation, they will often react with agitation or anxiety when caregivers convey frustration, irritation, anger, or rejection. Cuizon-Saiz (1988) provides a pertinent example below.

Mrs. X., a middle aged woman with Alzheimer's disease, would frequently become extremely agitated. She would clench her fists, scream, and run blindly down the hallways of the facility. In her terror, she would sometimes run into things or hit whatever, or whomever, was in her path. The staff found that if they called her name calmly and soothingly she would slow down. When her nonverbal behavior indicated the panic was subsiding, staff would hold her hand, rub her back, hug her, and she would sob her frustrations. When she was quiet, she would be assisted in a pleasant activity. In this case, even though the patient could not verbally express her needs, the staff were able, through trial and error, to learn the most satisfactory approach. Staff felt more effective and Mrs. X's periods of panic were forestalled or brief.

As previously stated, the first step in dealing with a patient with Alzheimer's disease is to explore the accuracy of the diagnosis. Sulkava, Haltia, Paetau, Wilkstrom, and Paolo (1983) have shown that as many as 18% of patients carefully diagnosed as having primary degenerative dementia did not show on autopsy the pathologic changes characteristic of Alzheimer's disease.

Because there is no cure for Alzheimer's disease, treatment success must be measured by reduction in symptoms and sequelae (Reifler, 1986). However, operating under the presumption that nothing can be done because a cure is not available would be entirely false (Reifler, Larson, Featherstone, & Cox, 1981). Almost one third of Alzheimer's patients have shown improvement in cognitive or physical abilities, or in "activities of daily living" when treated for coexisting medical illnesses or psychiatric problems. Examples of treatable problems include depression, overmedication, hypothyroidism, congestive heart failure, and paranoia. There are often treatable components or symptoms in the presence of irreversible dementias. Reifler (1986) believes that agitation is an indicator of poor prognosis in Alzheimer's disease and speculates that these patients may have coexisting Parkinson's disease. This would be a reason to seriously examine the use of major tranquilizers that are notorious for exacerbating symptoms of Parkinson's.

Psychotic symptoms can be expected to occur in the course of Senile Dementia of the Alzheimer's Type (SDAT). Rubin, Devverts, and Burke (1987) identified the following symptoms in a longtitudinal study of persons with Alzheimer's disease:

Paranoid delusions	30%
Misidentification of persons on TV and in mirrors	23%
Visual hallucinations	24%
Systematized delusions	4%

Accurate description of psychotic symptoms will assist in evaluating the appropriateness and therapeutic efficacy of treatments.

Symptoms of SDAT are often seen as predictable and progressive. However, Vanthooft (1987) disagrees with these assumptions and proposes that the behavior of demented persons involves personality traits that mediate the response to the losses involved. Prior personality disorders, levels of basic trust, and physical disorders all impinge on the demonstrated response to the primary defects experienced. In addition, the care of nursing home patients with SDAT where activity and ambulation is stressed appears to reduce need for tranquilizing medications. Vanthooft also concluded that rapid deterioration is not inescapable in a nursing home setting that is attendant to psychosocial needs.

One aged man, a professor emeritus of a well-known university, has been successfully taking care of his afflicted wife for several years. She, like he, was a university professor and he found it most difficult to cope with the loss of her intellectual companionship. He has solved this problem well by hiring university students to care for her several hours a day which provides respite for him as well as intellectual stimulation.

Shomaker (1987) interviewed family members of Alzheimer's disease victims to find out about their past interest and behaviors. Apparently, the frequency and intensity of past behaviors increased while the expression of these often became inappropriate. Understanding of life patterns, however, can lead to making provision for their expression and to clearer understanding of what certain behaviors may signify. This study suggests that there is a relationship between premorbid behaviors and those demonstrated in the illness. Early stages of the disease were characterized by accentuation in both frequency and intensity of previous traits. Examples from this study included the following:

Wandering did not appear to be aimless. Men tried to return to their jobs after lunch, women tried to clean up or to go out shopping; some were looking for something that had been forgotten. In other words, the wandering did not seem to be aimless but rather an expression of earlier purposeful activity. For instance, those individuals who had engaged in an active life style were more prone to hyperactivity and wandering. Care plans might include more activity, such as walking or dancing, to decrease the need for inappropriate activity.

Hyperactivity was exhibited in compulsive, disorganized activities. Some patients became preoccupied with past sports, jobs, or hobbies. A bus driver was quiet only when he sat in the family car parked in front of the house.

Individuals who had always been very communicative tended to continue to be so even though their verbosity was often a collection of fragmented comments, cliches, and arguments. The family reported that the patients began to tell stories that were untrue. In some cases, this was undoubtedly confabulation. Individuals who had been very attentive to personal hygiene often spent time gazing in the mirror or seemed to have excessive concern for personal appearance. These needs can be recognized and augmented. Until the very latest stages of the disease, these persons would wear jewelry and cologne and try to arrange their hair.

Those who had always been somewhat emotional found it hard to control outbursts of emotion. Some outbursts of anger were in response to tactless persons discussing the patient's condition in their presence with the mistaken belief that they were incompetent to understand. Emotions, such as self-pity, affection, and generosity, seemed to be intensified by the disease process. Individuals who must emote may be encouraged to expend their emotional outbursts at particular times and directed toward events rather than other patients. One man seemed to evidence a total personality change which, upon further investigation, emerged when he was given Ritalin.

Working with an elderly person who has a dementing disorder can be extremely frustrating and nongratifying for caregivers. It is too easy to discount his or her humanity if there are no responses to confirm it. Despite this, caregivers best demonstrate their human compassion and hope by their manner of interacting with such difficult patients. Only by confronting and coping with such challenges can caregivers confirm their potential for personal growth and higher levels of development.

In this regard, Brauer (1987) presents a profile of the ideal caregiver of the demented aged. Characteristics were based upon the need for the patient to maintain a consistent sense of self, to modulate affectual expressions, to express needs effectively, and to use knowledge of the past and future hopes to mediate present experience. Since these capacities are all eroded to some extent, it is the caregiver who either assists or ignores the patient's attempts toward personal integration. The ideal caregiver is one who:

Is not threatened by the psychological changes occurring for the patient.
Can facilitate effective communication by understanding the patient's increasingly tenuous connection with the phenomenal world.
Can use the relationship to strengthen the patient's sense of self.

To accomplish these goals, a facility must provide staff training programs with didactic education, self-awareness, exercises, ongoing supervision, and support groups.

O'Connor (1985) has developed a particularly useful *Nurse's Self Assessment Guide* which provides a consciousness-raising exercise to examine caregiver ability to relate to patients with organic dementias (see below).

NURSE'S SELF-ASSESSMENT GUIDE

Do I avoid a client unless I have a specific task?
Do I talk to client or do I carry out procedures in silence?
Do I address the client by name?

Do I proceed with care in spite of client's objection?
Do I feed the client mechanically and hurry to finish?
Do I speak loudly even when there is no hearing problem?
Do I routinely assign this person to someone else if possible?
Do I recognize this client as having any strengths?
Do I consider ways to help the client understand the situation?
Do I instruct this client as I would any other with the hope that they will understand?
How do I feel about this client and his or her situation?
Do I feel the family has abandoned the client and, if so, why should I care?
Do I feel the family is unreasonable in their demands to assuage their guilt?
Do I ignore the family and their involvement with the client?
Do I feel the family is not managing decisions related to the client in a realistic manner?

Adapted from O'Connor (1985)

Despite the rather negative approach to this self-awareness tool, it could be quite easily converted to a positive approach by asking "When have you . . ." as opposed to "Do you . . ." In either case, it is a useful tool for examining the significance of the manner in which care is approached.

Zachow's (1984) work with a very old lady (Helen) with dementia who constantly repeated "wa, wa, wa, wa," in a loud voice was mentioned in Chapter 5. A common and significant problem of communication in demented persons is their seeming inability to control these meaningless verbal perseverations. However, Zachow assumed that Helen *wanted* to communicate. This may be the first and most important assumption. She also determined that there must be a way to reach through the gray shroud of emotional chaos that afflicts such patients. Her method was planned multisensorial stimulation daily for six weeks. She used touch, talk, Baroque music, body movement, and a combination of validation and fantasy to give meaning to all of Helen's actions. With continued work, Helen was eventually able to feed herself and to speak a few understandable words.

Because dementias are believed to result in disturbances of biorhythmicity exhibited in continuous babbling, sleep pattern disturbance, and basal metabolic rate disturbances, success of interventions may be based on restoration of biorhythmicity. It is also possible that select music has the potential for restoration of body rhythm. The ancient Greeks and Egyptians gave full credence to the therapeutic power of music. Caregivers have yet to seriously study the use of music with demented persons. Replications of Zachow's (1984) study are needed.

When caregivers can feel the continuum of life and death, youth and age, wisdom and impetuousness as all a part of themselves, it will no longer be difficult for them to relate to the fearful and dark side of human nature. Attaining compassion and love as the highest achievement in caregiving is a goal to be strived for. Beyond that there is only technology.

Pseudodementias

Ancill (1986, pp. 16–19) describes *pseudodementias* as consisting of four categories. Briefly, they include:

- *Depressive illness* that occurs in patients whose reserves of neuronal function are low. This may also overlay an organic dementia thus making it difficult to discriminate. The determinant is often the degree of response to antidepressant medication.
- *Ganser syndrome* in which a patient can carry out ADL's and comprehend questions but answers are off target. There seems to be some fluctuation in levels of ability and consciousness and often either a basically low IQ or an underlying hysterical personality. Satir (1972) would call this person a "distractor."
- *Psychotic pseudodementia* is observed in older folk who have a long history of mania or schizophrenia. The presentation of dementia is not uncommon but is episodic and usually of abrupt onset.
- *Organic pseudodementias* are all those systemic disorders that present with acute dementia. Delirium usually accompanies the disorder and a fluctuating level of consciousness is characteristic. Major categorical systems of pseudodementia likelihood are: drugs, endocrine, cardiac, respiratory, renal, gastrointestinal, nutritional, hematological, and inflammatory.

Interestingly, 40 elderly patients with pseudodementia were intensively treated for depression with alleviation of symptoms and restoration of intellectual functioning. In a longitudinal study of these persons by Kral and Emery (1987) it was found that 89% had eventually developed senile dementia of the Alzheimer's type. This study raises two questions of significance that need investigation:

(1) Is depressive dementia the first, although temporary, manifestation of SDAT? (2) Can major depressions or temporary cognitive impairment predispose one to the development of SDAT?

DEPRESSION

Depression is the foremost and most frequent problem of aged individuals. Propensity toward depression is thought to be on an organic basis and related to the decrease of neurotransmitter production in the brain. In addition, old age is a time of more losses than gains and each of these compounds to make depression an inevitability of late life. This is not meant to indicate that old age does not have many joys and rewards but only that depression must be anticipated at certain times. Thus, the most predictive element of a reasonable old age is in an individual's capacity to tolerate bouts of depression.

Statistics vary widely on the presence of depression in later life—estimates range anywhere from 20 to 70%. Reasons for this variance reside in the definition of depression, whether it is a primary or secondary diagnosis, and the overlap of vegetative symptoms normally apparent in late life that are indices of depression in young adulthood. In addition, persons diagnosed with dementia are often actually suffering profound depression.

Characteristics of Depression

Depression in old age is characterized by dysphoric affect, feelings of helplessness, hopelessness, and worthlessness accompanied by physical complaints of headache, insomnia, and extreme fatigue. As the depression deepens, memory impairment is common. Profound depression may also mimic dementia as the individual's social skills, judgment, and grooming deteriorate. The expressed desire to die is frequent and negative thoughts become ruminative. For elderly males suffering depression, the risk of suicide is extremely high. There are some indications that refusal to eat is a more passive method of suicide used by old women though statistics do not reflect this. In order to demonstrate the characteristics of depression across the age span, Table 6.4 presents a comparative chart.

Helplessness

Exaggerated helplessness may be the reaction of an elder to increasing disability or the caregiver's awareness of the elder's diminished abil-

TABLE 6.4 Depression across Life Span

Characteristics	Child	Young Adult	Middle Aged	Old
	Hyperactive	Unpredictable	Females most vulnerable	Lethargy
	Accident prone	Impulsive	Apathy	Confusion
	Hyperphagia or	Subliminal suicide	Vegetative signs	Poverty of thought
	Anorexia	Violence	More often disabling or	Irritability
	School phobia	Substance abuse	psychotic	Hostility
		Sexual promiscuity		Hypochondria
		Anorexia		
Precipitants	Interruption in attachment	Interpersonal conflict	Spiritual conflicts	Real deprivation
	Bereavement	Unemployment	Ennui	Multiple losses
	Abuse	School failure	Anomie	Physiologic changes
	Gain or loss of sibling	Broken love affairs	Empty nest	Relocation
		Loneliness	Illness	Retirement
		Leaving parental home	Signs of aging	Illness
			Meaninglessness	Impaired function
Coping	Regression	Blaming	Regression	Denial
Strategies	Overcompensation	Sublimation	Withdrawal	Projection
	Rejection	Challenging	Projection	Dependency
		Suicidual gestures	Psychosomatic illness	Regression suicide
				Compulsions
				Paranoia/guarded
Therapies most	Play therapy	Peer groups	Psychotherapy groups	Suicide prevention
comonly used	Surrogate caregivers	Individual counseling	Drugs	Drugs
	Drugs-Ritalin	Cognitive restructuring	Career counseling	Life-review
	Parental counseling	Stress reduction	Electro-convulsive therapy	Remotivation groups
		Group living situations	Life-review	Reminiscence
		Crisis hot lines		

193

ity. The insecurity engendered may accentuate neediness and dependency and further threaten the caregiving relationship. Counseling should address the maintenance of maximum functional capacity, perhaps some *benign* neglect, while attending to the motivation underlying the phenomenon and encouraging expression of feelings of the elder and the caregiver in conjoint sessions.

Multiple Complaints and Demands

The patient who continually complains and makes demands on the staff or family is often merely expressing his or her depression. Caregivers tend to recognize that hypochondriasis is a thermometer of depression in the old; they can measure fulmination of depression by increase in body preoccupation. Unfortunately, caregivers are not so inclined to see the demanding and complaining client as also depressed. Unfounded complaints, such as "He never brought me the newspaper he promised," "She never remembers to bring my pain medication on time," or "No one ever listens to me" are particularly difficult for the staff. If caregivers hear the underlying message, however, it is almost always one of struggling against feelings of worthlessness and helplessness. Since such behavior can lead to overuse of medication, staff annoyance, or staff avoidance, it is a legitimate target for intervention. According to Hussian (1986), it is also possible that a history of unfounded complaints may lead caregivers to ignore a reasonable request.

In addition, it is important to rule out an organic cause prior to instituting a behavioral intervention, such as extinction. The classic symptoms of a disease process may be absent or different among the elderly; therefore, one should consider that the complaints stem from a reality base until it becomes clear that they are based in depression and hypochondriasis. If the frequency of complaints is extremely high, there is no evidence of a physical disorder, and the client also complains frequently about nonsomatic issues, the staff may safely assume it is evidence of depression. The resulting intervention should be designed to build small, pleasurable events into the daily schedule, ignore unreasonable complaints, and foster discussion with the client on the presence of depression. The caregiver may even need to remind the client periodically, "Remember, we talked about these feelings of neglect and discomfort as being symptoms of your depression."

In order not to reinforce the complaining behavior, Hussian (1986) has suggested the following actions:

Fix attention away from the client who is complaining
Do not make a verbal or nonverbal response
If the behavior becomes frustrating the observer should turn away
and leave the room

Cuizon-Saiz (1988) provides an example of a successful intervention.

> Mrs. N. had severe osteoarthritis, pain, and depression. She was very demand-
> ing and consumed an inordinate amount of staff time yet they were never able
> to please her. A staff meeting was called to decide how to deal with this difficult
> lady. The nursing assistants decided they would provide personal care for
> Mrs. N at a regular time each morning and make her as comfortable as possible.
> They would inform her of the exact time they would be back to meet any of her
> other needs. When they were late, they would give an apology and an explana-
> tion. They checked her every two hours. When she began to feel secure with
> this regime and realized that she would be attended to consistently, her demands
> began to decrease.

Berezin (1983) poses an interesting idea in relation to complaining
and its possible relationship to depression. From his perspective, it
may be dynamically useful for the elderly to complain. The compul-
sive/obsessive person uses projection as a major defense mechanism.
Blaming others for unhappiness serves to prevent him or her from
internalizing the problem and blaming him or herself. In this way, his
or her defense protects him or her from being overwhelmed and, at
times, from suicide.

Anxiety and Depression

In a study by Rabins (1987), while younger depressives reported
more episodes of anxiety than elder depressives, elder depressives
were more likely to be judged hypochondriacal. In another study,
Kretschmar and Wurthmann (1987) found those with agitated depression were most likely to make slow progress toward recovery.
Mintzer, D'Elia, Mintz, Small, and Jarvik (1987) found symptoms of
anxiety and depression were closely related in geriatric patients and
observed a high correlation over time. Improvement in either of the
symptoms was predictive of improvement in the other. In cases where
anxiety is a major feature of depression, Dehlin et al. (1987) recommend Alprazolam be prescribed in dosages of 0.5 to 3.0 mgm daily.
This benzodiazepine is effective in the treatment of anxiety accompanied by depression and is judged far safer for elders than the more
commonly prescribed tricyclic antidepressants.

Age and Gender

Age and gender differences in sociomedical correlates of depression were identified by Husaini, Linn, Nesser, Whitten-Stouzl, and Miller (1987). Persons over 61 years of age suffering from higher levels of depression tended to report low ego strength, poor health, few confidants, and lower levels of social support than persons suffering depression at younger ages. Male and female differences emerged as well: depression among males was exacerbated by poor health; depression in females was affected by a lower, or less satisfactory, support system.

Patterns of Depression

A study of patterns of depression among women in late life revealed three major recurring themes (Wasson & Grunes, 1987):

Trapped and angry: resentful of their inclination to put other's needs before their own
Anxious and lonely: responses to widowhood and social losses
Valueless and despairing: illness and incapacity had undermined their sense of independence and control.

Poststroke depression is clearly correlated with degree of functional and intellectual impairment. Using the Beck rating scale, over 50% of poststroke subjects rated themselves as significantly depressed. There seemed to be no relationship between the severity of depression and left versus right hemispheric brain injury.

Reactive Depression

Patients with medical illnesses are frequently subject to secondary depressions related to disease processes. Borson (1987) found that patients with chronic obstructive pulmonary disease (COPD) are particularly vulnerable to depression. The depression is often accompanied by anxiety and panic. All symptoms were found responsive to tricyclic therapy.

Talbot (1987) studied reactive depression related to residing in a nursing home. Findings from this study indicate a direct correlation between depth of depression and length of time residing in a nursing home.

Elderly depressed persons generally experience longer duration of the disorder, clustered episodes, a tendency toward chronicity, and poorer response to medication. In addition, they are more inclined to demonstrate cognitive impairment as a symptom of depression. Given this knowledge, it behooves caregivers to seek creative methods of dealing with this most prevalent problem of elderly patients.

Assisting a client to measure his or her level of depression may be the first step toward instituting a measure of control and involvement in recovery. Beck and Beck (1972) has developed a brief scale for such an activity called "A Step Ladder of Depression." Clients seem willing to participate in evaluating their depression and sometimes express relief that it is not rated as severe as they had thought (see Table 6.5).

Gurland (in Liptzin, 1986) noted that aged depressed persons tend to see their physicians often but receive little specific antidepressant treatment. Most often they are given tranquilizers, which may actually exacerbate the problem. Teeter (in Liptzin, 1986) studied 74 patients in two nursing homes and identified primary depression in more than one fourth and secondary depression in almost one half of the sample. Bettis (1979), Gallagher (1983), Gurland (1976), and others have shown the prevalence of depression as a major problem of the aged. Findings indicate that older patients frequently present with depression so profound it mimics dementia and has thus been classified as pseudodementia. The diagnosis is generally made by exclusion when no organic pathology can be found. Additionally, trials of antidepressants may be useful though there are high nonresponse rates even in clearcut depressive illnesses. In the absence of clear cut diagnosis, criteria described by Wells (1982) have been useful as a screening measure. In addition, Sakauye (1986) has identified social withdrawal, global errors of omission, acuteness of onset, past psychiatric history, and the tendency of the patient to point out errors rather than hiding them as all suggestive of a depressive pseudodementia.

Depression may result from the absence of positive reinforcement by others, rewards that are unrelated to behavior, and reinforcement that is appropriate but infrequent. It becomes apparent that some common ways of dealing with the elderly may not only reinforce unwanted behaviors but deepen depression. For instance, when John fondles his genitals openly in the day room, he usually receives attention from the staff, negative though it may be. Sometimes he is quickly hustled off to play bingo; at other times, the staff simply ignores the behavior. Once in a long while, an enlightened staff person will talk directly to him about his sexuality and the appropriateness of masturbating in private. Families, or significant others, can play an important role and need to be involved in any efforts toward behavior modification. John, for example, will need touching and caring ges-

TABLE 6.5   Beck Depression Inventory, Short Form

1. I feel that the future is hopeless and that things cannot improve.
   I feel I have nothing to look forward to.
   I feel discouraged about the future.
   I am not particularly pessimistic or discouraged about the future.
2. I feel I am a complete failure as a person (parent, husband, wife).
   As I look back on my life, all I can see is a lot of failures.
   I feel I have failed more than the average person.
   I do not feel like a failure.
3. I feel as though I am very bad or worthless.
   I feel quite guilty.
   I feel bad or unworthy a good part of the time..
   I don't feel particularly guilty.
4. I hate myself.
   I am disgusted with myself.
   I am disappointed in myself.
   I don't feel disappointed in myself.
5. I have lost all of my interest in other people and don't care about them at all.
   I have lost most of my interest in other people and have little feeling for them.
   I am less interested in other people than I used to be.
   I have not lost interest in other people.
6. I can't make any decisions at all anymore.
   I have great difficulty in making decisions.
   I try to put off making decisions.
   I make decisions as well as ever.
7. I feel that I am ugly or repulsive-looking.
   I feel that there are permanent changes in my appearance and they make me look
      unattractive.
   I don't feel that I look any worse than I used to.
8. I get too tired to do anything.
   I get tired from doing anything.
   I get tired more easily than I used to.
   I don't get any more tired than usual.

Each question is weighted in rank order from 1 to 4 pts. Total cumulative points:
0–4   = No depression present.
5–7   = Mild depression, able to function; will lift in a few weeks.
8–15 = Moderate depression, able to function with difficulty; help from professionals highly
         recommended.
16+   = Severe depression, must have professional help.

Adapted from Beck Depression Inventory, Short Form. Beck, A., & Beck, R. (1972). Screening depressed patients in family practice: A rapid technique. *Postgraduate Medicine*, vol. 52, pp. 83–84. Reprinted with permission.

tures from family members on a continuing basis. He will also need to be assured that his sexuality is recognized even though institutional living may make it difficult to express.

Yet another reason for depression is loss of personal effectiveness. In nursing homes, often ineffective behaviors are those that are noticed while individual strengths and resources are seldom identified, much less reinforced. Through discussion and observation, each resident should have areas of personal effectiveness documented. Opportunities for expressing these strengths and for recognition need to be built into daily schedules. Often, this is done informally but not consistently and positive reinforcement may be lacking. In addition, activities undertaken by the elder should have meaning and not be just a way of keeping him or her busy. Conceivably, institutions could document cost benefits by carefully using the talents of individuals. I have often heard the argument that management is not allowed to make the residents work. This is a superficial and trite dismissal. Obviously, there are ways to use an individual's skills without abusing them. A modified sheltered workshop model with particular rewards for participation might be instituted. Individuals might then be paired to pool their skills when one is incapable of accomplishment without assistance.

Mobilizing the Depressed Client

As the sense of helplessness becomes internalized and experienced as self-failure, the individual becomes convinced of failure in any activity undertaken. Thus, he or she is reluctant to do anything. A gradual return to effectiveness can be accomplished using the five steps identified by Manderino and Bzdek (1986) shown below.

> *Balance rest and activity:* Mutually structure a schedule of rest periods and activity periods. Every hour of the day should be carefully plotted. Caregiver should discuss the physiologic benefits of interspersed rest and activity.
>
> *Supervise activity:* Invite client's participation in an activity in which he or she cannot fail (such as making a collage). If client refuses, validity of reasons should be evaluated and discussed specifically and counteracted realistically. Activity will then be scheduled for a little later or new activity devised. To be dynamically useful, all of this must be done in a warm and nonjudgmental manner. It is more important for the client to make an attempt than to succeed. Avoidance of interpretations of failure is most significant. Discuss the fact that *it is alright not to succeed* and that trying is most important. Failure to succeed must not be interpreted as further inability as it will reinforce the negative cycle of despondency.
>
> *Retrieval of pleasure and mastery.* Clients may have forgotten pleasurable activities. Assist them to keep a daily log of

anything that produces momentary pleasure and of each activity mastered throughout the day. Ask that they rate degrees of satisfaction from 1 through 5, so even small gains can be measured.

Client will be encouraged and assisted to construct a list of all things in the past that have given enjoyment. This may be a difficult task as depressed persons are inclined to forget pleasurable aspects of life. From this list, certain pleasurable events can be built into the daily schedule.

An example of such a care plan follows. It will take additional staff time to implement the plan but should result in greater participation and an overall time saving.

DAILY REST AND ACTIVITY SCHEDULE

8:00 Arise, wash face, brush teeth, and comb hair.
8:30 Eat breakfast.
9:00 Attend community meeting. Not expected to speak.
9:30 Rest in room.
10:30 Dress for lunch.
11:30 Eat lunch.
12:30 Rest in room.
1:30 Phone a family member or friend.
2:00 Attend a music group.
3:00 Rest in room.
4:00 Join others in lounge for tea.
5:00 Eat dinner.
6:00 Rest in room.
7:00 Listen to news on radio or TV.
8:00 Prepare for bed with warm bath.
9:00 Accept gentle foot or back massage from nurse.
9:30 Retire.

The importance of frequent discussion, supervision, and encouragement of the client must be stressed. The client should have a copy of the schedule and indicate which things were particularly hard to accomplish and which gave some satisfaction. Remember, success will be realized in small gradients and erratic patterns; it's O.K. for the client not to succeed; progress must be discussed and carefully monitored.

Asking the client to identify everything done last week that was difficult reassures him or her that the caregiver knows he or she is having a hard time. In addition, it may be useful to encourage the client to identify events that stimulate feelings of sadness, times of day when he or she feels most depressed, and anything that produces feelings of fear and anxiety. It is important to balance the emphasis on negative aspects of depression with something positive.

A group of depressed elders in a day care center constructed the following list of things that have, in the past, given them pleasure. The group mode may be used with depressed persons if it does not entail any elements of competition.

Piano playing.
Tea.
Reading the Bible.
Listening to opera.
Sexual activity.
Walking.
Buying fresh flowers.
Writing letters to friends.
Reading poetry.
Buying a new dress.
Baking cookies.
Stringing beads.
Traveling.
Sharing war stories with other veterans.
Doing things with grandchildren.

When a group of clients really begin to think about what they have enjoyed, such lists can be endless. In addition, most items can be adapted to various care settings.

For instance, several facilities of which I am aware have instituted "travel days." One of them, Benedictine Nursing Center in Mt. Angel, Oregon, recently had "A Day in Ireland." Staff involved the surrounding community in making special foods, costumes, activities, and loaning items from Ireland to the facility for a day. Green beer was provided with a dinner of corned beef and cabbage. The occupational therapy room was converted to a simulated torture chamber. Horse races were broadcast over the intercom. Staff were dressed like Irish maids and men. Lephrechauns were visible in various places. Irish dancers gave a performance in the evening. A small simulated castle was set up in one storage room where a princess waited to tell fortunes. The residents were caught up in the excitement

202   Caring for the Psychogeriatric Client

of the event and contributed any skills they had toward making it successful. Individuals from the community involved in the planning visited the facility and interacted with the residents. For names of other facilities see resources.

Hallinger (1986) found that, when touch was applied in a gentle and caring manner, increased frequency and duration of verbal communication was demonstrated among depressed elders. Though this seems entirely logical and concepts of "therapeutic touch" have been accepted for more than two decades, caregivers sometimes neglect to apply them.

Group Restoration of Effectiveness

When the depressed individual has progressed to lesser levels of debilitation, group participation becomes a successful mode of intervention. To this date, numerous types of groups have been used with varying degrees of client improvement in morale and socialization. Ebersole (1979, 1981), Ostrovski (1980), Parsons (1986), Wichita (1977), and many others have used reminiscence activities as a topical vehicle for groups of depressed persons. All reported significant success in lifting of depression as well as other gains, such as increased levels of attention, appetite, and social interaction. However, it is important to mention that other results have not been positive (Boylin, Gordon, & Nerke, 1976). The consistency, continuity over time, and discrimination regarding the activation of "life-review" must be given careful consideration before activating such group activities (see Chapter 5 for further suggestions for group activities). Group activities may involve many nonverbal and pleasureable activities that derive additional meaning when shared with a few selected individuals. The following brief descriptions of such activities is meant to serve as a springboard for individual ideas.

Reminiscing to Alleviate Depression   Ostrovski (1980) began a reminiscing group with depressed elders in a mental health day care center and found it successful in promoting client interaction and in elevating morale. Shared memories are individual and do not promote a competitive spirit or the need to focus on failure. A group leader must structure such groups toward events that were likely to have given pleasure, such as first jobs, family rituals, special foods enjoyed in childhood, favorite teacher, and other events. Parsons (1986) reports on a reminiscing group with depressed persons in which depression was significantly alleviated after six weeks. She also found participants focused attention better, interacted more socially, and, by sharing, assuaged some painful feelings. Two cautions are important with such groups, however: do not allow group members to bog down the group with examples of personal failures; the filter of the current depression is likely to skew their remembrances and they should be made aware of this. (See Chapter 4 for additional discussion of reminiscing.)

Body Awareness Developing body awareness is a critical element in the development of health perception and wellness orientation. A creative method for developing body awareness was done by a senior citizen's group who wrote poems about offending body parts and then published them as a group (Boise Seniors, 1983). My example when using this process is provided below:

My Heart
I can   Feel
My heart is big and thumps along
As it carries life to obscure worlds
Each cell a universe its own
So faithfully served
By my old
Heart

The heart is a circus calliope singing.

A life-force pulses through its tubes, valves, chambers.

We marvel at the simplicity of its action, the sustaining vitality of its function.

Its sound is unmistakable—akin to no other.

Companion to our mood, it sighs and soars, harmonizing mood with beat and measure throughout life's parade.

And when its song ends, the silence is

a

   b

       s

           o

               l

                   u

                       t

                           e.

BOB HAGER

Source: Boise Council on Aging, Boise, ID. Now My Soul Has Elbow Room, 1983. Permission to use has been granted.

In the beginning
I was first to form
A tiny metronome
A supreme regulator of
Life's precious fluid.

Excelerating to Passion's call
"Love You With All My Heart"
Slowing to Sorrow's blast
"You're Breaking My Heart"
A center of emotions.

Continuing the appointed task
Following the Master Plan
Earthly assignments fulfilled
Beating out life's last fleeting breath
The human heart at rest.
                                                THELMA BECK

Source: Boise Council on Aging, Boise, ID. Now My Soul Has Elbow Room, 1983.
Permission to use has been granted.

In addition to constructing visual and poetic metaphors about
the body, therapeutic touch, self-massage, and movement expressive of musical passages can bring one into harmony with the sensual aspects of body. Such awareness will aid the elder in shifting
perception of the body as a source of pain, discomfort, and betrayal.
Also, while younger persons may be quite comfortable with body
awareness activities, elders may have thought of them, if at all, as
fads of youth. For elders, however, this subconscious relegation of
certain activities to youth may work to their advantage when re-
introduced slowly and in a nonthreatening manner. For example,
begin with a self-massage of the hand or foot, later add music
and a rhythmic movement to the massage. Scented lotion appeals
to yet another sense. The multisensorial impact can add to the
enjoyment of the experience in elders who have some loss of sensory
acuity.

When the group has become secure and demonstrates comfort with
a technique or activity, add a new dimension. Choreograph movement with music and wands, fans or hoops. Elders can be taught to
follow a leader in unison movements or can be given free expression.
In either case, the enjoyment of body motion stimulated by movement has the additional advantage of providing range of motion
exercises without becoming an onerous task for the individual or the
staff.

Identifying Earlier Coping Responses   In the process of surviving to old age, elders have developed sophisticated coping skills. When they are feeling helpless or discouraged, it may be necessary to help them identify their coping skills more specifically. For instance, Marge often worked her frustrations out while gardening; Mabel went shopping; Miriam would sing at the top of her lungs; Jean would tell her cat all of her troubles; Carol would call her friends; and Georgia would make an entry in her journal. Each individual has developed distinctive ways of coping with discouraging or frustrating events, ways that externalize the attendant anxiety (Martens, 1986). Some have also internalized feelings or relied on unhealthy habits such as overeating, drinking, or brooding. Safe to say, most have a range of healthy and unhealthy coping skills. In all cases, however, the goal is to identify and intensify the use of the healthy adaptive skills and diminish reliance on abdication, apathy, and hopelessness.

Behavioral Approaches to Alleviating Depression   Depression is likely to result from sudden situational changes in which previous rewards are no longer available and rewards of the new situation have not yet been discovered. Because one has not had the opportunity to contemplate the new situation, suddenness of the change may be a significant factor. The most extreme example of this might be seen when an elderly widow, immediately following the death of her spouse, is moved to the home of her daughter. Obviously, there will be many losses and deep depression. However, with careful planning and time to consider her decision before moving, the widow may decide that living with her daughter may provide pleasures that she is not able to achieve on her own. Occasionally, it is fruitful, particularly for one inclined to compulsive behavior, to construct lists of positives and negatives to be found in the new situation.

When examining the reward systems an individual has established or is seeking, it is critical to respond by modifying the environment as well as the individual's expectations. Thus, when an individual moves into a nursing home, and begins to participate in group activities, it is incumbent on facility management to adapt to the individual just as the individual must adapt to the environment. Unfortunately, this is seldom done.

Cognitive-Behavioral Therapy   Beck, Rush, Shaw, and Emery's (1979) cognitive-behavioral therapy was developed specifically for depressive states. Yost, Beutler, Corbishley, and Allender (1986) have adapted this to work with groups of depressed elders. As such, it is particularly applicable to long-term care facilities. Because of its specificity, it is also usable by personnel who have little background in psychodynamics.

The unique effects of cognitive therapy on self-concept, perceptions of personal control, and diminished feeling of hopelessness make cognitive-behavioral therapy particularly useful in the treatment of depression in the elderly.

Correcting irrational attitudes is fundamental to changing pathological feelings and behaviors. Such attitudes as, "Nothing matters," "I can't do anything right," "This is what I deserve," "I'm too old to try it," "Life was so much better in the old days," "I'm just waiting to die," are particular cognitive distortions common to the aged. Germinated by ageism, the unfairness of life, and the realities of failing capacities, these all have a kernel of truth. Because they are not totally false perceptions, society and caregivers are prone to accept such attitudes without critical examination. However, this tendency toward "all or none" thinking must be interrupted by a dialectic process, which is precisely the advantage of a group over a one-on-one approach in which the therapist has not yet personally experienced the impact of old age. In a group of elders, each can modify the perception of the others. In addition, the leader must not allow the group to bog down in depressive monologues but keep to the task. For example, the leader may write on a blackboard each of the members' attitudes about their life at present and then have the group discuss each one in depth.

Following the initial phases of group development (getting acquainted, understanding the purpose of the group, and developing beginning trust and interest in the group), it is suitable to establish reasonable individual goals. What would make each individual feel better? What would each like to accomplish? Some want to "be like my old self again." What is it about that "old self" that they miss the most? How do they measure when they feel better? Group members must be helped to be specific. Refining global statements and assisting group members to set small measurable activities will be indices of progress. For example, the wish to be "like my old self" can be refined to "I want to sleep better at night." Then one must assist in identifying means of measuring better sleep; perhaps gradually waking less or staying awake for shorter periods. Then one must identify the rituals or situations that have produced good sleep and begin to implement them one by one. Of course, there will be times when no apparent progress is made. As previously stated, it is essential these not be interpreted as failures. Responses such as "It didn't work, I hardly slept at all!" or "I knew it wouldn't work" could be countered with "Perhaps you tried too hard" or "Maybe we can try another method or perhaps it is best to wait a few days. You may need to allow yourself time to think about this." Or, "What is it about not sleeping that really worries you?"

These brief suggestions are a beginning point for group cognitive therapy. Depending on the capacities of the members involved, there are numerous intricacies that can be employed. For more extensive application refer to the cited work of Yost et al.

SUICIDE

Suicide among males remains a problem of the highest incidence in late life but the potential danger is much less frequently discussed or considered in relation to the aged client than with those who are younger. Figure 6.1 presents a comparison of suicide rates by age, race, and sex.

Suicide in the elderly varies with sex, age, and geographical location. Women most often suffered depression whereas men were most motivated toward suicide by physical illness. In rural locations, suicide was accomplished through "hard" methods such as shooting or hanging while in urban areas intoxication was a more frequent means (Haring, Miller, Barnas, Fleischacker, 1987). Women are most suicidal between ages 45 and 55 while men become increasingly more suicidal with age. In Japan, it has been noted that in certain situations an old woman will commit suicide because of a belief that she is no longer a useful member of the family and thus does not deserve to live (Kato, 1987).

Signs of suicidal intent may manifest differently in elders than in younger persons. When a young person begins to give significant personal belongings away, it is seen as a signal of potential suicide. Older persons do many things to bring closure to life, however. They may give things away, contact persons not seen in years, talk of death frequently, and even say they wish they could die, all of these without actual suicidal intent.

In general, however, suicide is the last and most obvious evidence of control one may evince. While the suicide rate doubles for men from youth to old age, the homicide rate remains approximately half that of youth. This could easily be interpreted as evidence that in late life one is more likely to internalize failure or problems than to blame it on others or conditions.

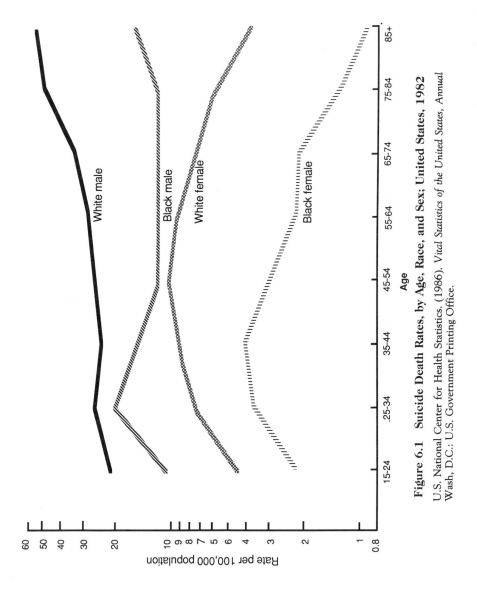

Figure 6.1 Suicide Death Rates, by Age, Race, and Sex: United States, 1982

U.S. National Center for Health Statistics. (1986). *Vital Statistics of the United States, Annual* Wash, D.C.: U.S. Government Printing Office.

Dynamics of Suicide in Aged Men

Aged Caucasian males have long been recognized as the most suicide prone persons in the United States. The longer they live, the more suicidal they become. The dynamic is commonly related to these causes: disappointment with one's life course; present deficits in physical capabilities; and unavailability of resources that provide sustenance and pleasure.

In addition, the core dynamic often manifests as *a sense of being out of control*. In a culture where men are socialized to take control of their own destinies, to captain their own ships, so to speak, it is a massive erosion of self-esteem to confront failure in those respects. Superimposed upon that is the unbearable shame felt when one is unable to control bodily functions. An example of the importance and pride in function was provided by an elderly gentleman in Tucson who refused to leave his apartment because he could no longer walk without the assistance of a cane. As he stated, "Oh, no, I couldn't go outside. You know, someone might see me, someone I know. A man has a sense of dignity, you know" (Hotchkiss, 1982).

Interestingly, the statistics bear out the fact that the more one feels the expectation or burden of success the more prone one is to suicide when not successful. Thus, blacks' suicide rate has risen as more expectations and opportunities have been made available to them.

Dynamics of Suicide in Mid-Life Women

For mid-life women, the principal dynamic of suicide manifests as a *diminished sense of self* in relation to others' needs and appraisal. In recent generations of mid-life women, the dynamic may be more related to feelings of being deprived of opportunities for personal development in their youth. Unfortunately, the impact of the feminist movement on the self-concept of women at mid-life has not been fully explored. Yet caregivers know that the suicide rate peaks for all women between the ages of 45 and 54. At that time women are:

- Confronted with evidences of aging.
- Experiencing changes in reproductive capacities.
- Concerned about loss of sexual attractiveness.
- No longer able to rationalize existence in terms of the activities of wife and mother.
- Feeling unprepared and unsupported in launching new careers or directions for self-development.

Many of our present elderly women had no opportunity to develop any sense of identity unrelated to family roles. In other words, their sense of self has been largely dependent on the appraisal of others: children, parents, husbands, and a sexist society. Relinquishment of such comfortable roles and patterns came when hormonal changes were also a factor that were reckoned with, although having completed the female mid-life adjustment they are usually no longer highly suicidal.

At this point, a significant question arises: Why do women end their lives more frequently during the mid-life crisis and men endure only to end their lives at a much later time? In purely practical terms, it would appear women have much more reason to end their lives in their later years:

- Half of retired elderly women are widowed and have an annual income of less than $5,000.
- Only 35% of women over 65 years are married.
- Most live alone.
- Many are relocated, to live with family members irrespective of their wishes, at the time of widowhood.
- They are far more likely to become victims of abuse and neglect than male elders in similar situations (Older American Reports, 1983).

Speculations are that women learn early to be more adaptable to imposed situations. They also learn some degree of gratification with household/family management tasks that provide a sense of meaningful activity. However repetitious and nondemanding such activities seem, they do provide a feeling of familiarity and security. Of course, even with mild to moderate degrees of impairment, these daily activities can be carried on. When residing with family or others, they may feel a sense of usefulness. Men, on the other hand, have to make considerably more effort to find such sustaining activities and more often must leave the security of the home to do so. In any case, they appear to feel worse in old age than women with similar situations.

Assessment of Suicide Potential

Suicide potential may have entirely different indications in the old. For instance, evidences of closure in relationships, giving away treasured articles, making a will, disengagement, and even statements of the desire for death may only be indications that the individual is working toward a satisfactory and meaningful death experience. This may, indeed, be a very mature and healthy activity.

Therefore, assessment of suicide potential must consist of the following:

- Skillful interviewing and listening to what is not said as well as what is said.
- Determining future events that seem to have meaning.
- Identifying losses that erode sense of competence.
- A review of recent history of accidents.
- Awareness that old women may starve themselves. Passive methods of suicide are not common in men.
- Defining marked changes in mood or life-style.

Below is a further listing of special factors to consider that increase suicidal potential.

FACTORS THAT INCREASE SUICIDAL POTENTIAL

Alienation: few close friends.
Limited interests in organizations or hobbies.
Experiencing chronic insomnia.
Depressed, ill, and in pain.
Reliance on drugs and alcohol.
Receiving extensive and painful medical treatment.
Withdrawal from usual areas of involvement.
Bereavement, especially loss of spouse.
Lingering illness with expectation of death.
Expressed feelings of helplessness and hopelessness.
Meaninglessness.
Decreased self-regard.
Functional and mental deterioration.

Planning Care of the Suicidal Elderly Male

The overall planned interventions for a suicidal elderly male must have an expected outcome of increased sense of control, self-esteem, self-sufficiency, and a meaning in remaining alive. Expanding the social contacts and social network without these specific end goals is likely to be unsuccessful. Marshall (1978) and Miller (1978) have shown that many male suicides were neither single nor alone.

Dealing with a Suicidal Client: A Sample Case

Bill was a 76-year-old retired executive who had taken great pride in his competence. Bill's myth was of imperviousness to the ordinary assaults of life. He believed he could manage in situations that others found intolerable. But, he also believed in intrinsic justice: a man got what he deserved. The community health nurse who visited Bill in his home as he was assimilating his recent diagnosis of bladder cancer found him extremely depressed. While she expected this, in discussing his diagnosis and expectations of what lay ahead she detected a serious disjuncture in his values and beliefs activated by his disease. He spoke of his intention to alter his life style in whatever way necessary to conquer the disease. However, this dynamic approach belied the obvious depressive affect he conveyed. The nurse understood his depression and sense of futility when he later said, "You know, the thing I can't make sense of is why this has happened to me. I have always lived carefully and not abused my body, myself, or the rights of others. I'm a fair man and this seems like a real injustice to me; something I didn't deserve and yet couldn't do anything to prevent." Suddenly it became clear to the nurse that his two myths were in conflict: his carefully planned life had not resulted in justice and reward and he clearly had lost control of it.

Once the nurse had identified the conflicting myths, her goal was to modify their meaning until Bill could accept it. While he alone could come to this resolution, the facilitative skills of the nurse could be instrumental in assisting him.

Her first concern was for the intensity of his depression. He had taken to his bed and not eaten, shaved, or bathed since he learned of his diagnosis four days ago. His wife was extremely upset by this uncharacteristic behavior. In addition, she was absorbed in her own incipient grief process with the beginning awareness that her strong, capable husband was vulnerable to the frailties of mankind.

The nurse realized the crisis they were in and made no attempt at that time to modify myths but only to bring some degree of physical and psychic comfort to the situation. Coupling her awareness of Bill's need to be strong and in control and finding the wife's ability to express concern about her mate's refusal to eat, the nurse approached Bill first to alter the situation in a positive direction. She was also aware that restoration of predictable patterns would be most useful when the world seemed to have gone awry. Had she not been perceptive, it is conceivable she could have attempted to have Bill hospitalized for dehydration or potential suicide. The spousal system that could restore balance would then be thrown into further chaos.

Specifically, the nurse talked to Bill about his wife's needs. Often, when one is depressed, one is unable to consider the needs of others, but here the nurse was counting on the sustaining strength of Bill's life-long pattern of taking action. While these kinds of interventions are somewhat of a gamble—human behavior being never totally predictable—the nurse knew the risk was minimal if the intervention proved ineffective. To illuminate this further, Table 6.6 presents a process recording of the nurse's therapeutic interaction with Bill.

Understanding the Conceptual Model   The following will explain the concepts that guided the nurse's interventions:

TABLE 6.6 Process Recording of Therapeutic Interaction with Bill

Nurse:	Bill, you are depressed and that is important for you right now. You need this time to retreat and reflect.
Bill:	I'm not depressed. I have never allowed myself that sort of indulgence.
Analysis:	Nurse is giving Bill permission to be less effective without erosion of his self-esteem. She recognized that he will probably not be able to immediately admit he is less than capable of handling this situation but that her statement may be used later as Bill tries to make sense of the situation.
Nurse:	I know you are not accustomed to self-indulgence. That is one reason you are able to handle this situation without completely falling apart.
Bill:	Well, I would like to just forget the whole thing and give up. It doesn't seem to matter much one way or the other.
Analysis:	Bill is expressing ambivalence and anger.
Nurse:	What have you thought about since you were told you had bladder cancer?
Bill:	Well, I thought about ending it all quick and cheap.
Nurse:	Do you mean you thought of killing yourself?
Analysis:	The nurse makes explicit the statement Bill may be reluctant to state.
Bill:	Well, certainly not to prolong the situation more than I must.
Nurse:	Meaning?
Bill:	If I don't eat, I think I'll probably only last about 40 days in this wilderness.
Analysis:	Bill is beginning to try to make sense out of his experience by equating it with Christ's experience in mortification of the flesh.
Nurse:	Sounds like Christ in the wilderness.
Bill:	No, I'm just being practical.
Nurse:	Are you concerned about lingering a long time in pain?
Analysis:	Nurse seeking clarification.
Bill:	Some, but I'm more concerned about becoming weak, pathetic, an object of pity and a burden to my wife. You know, most of us old codgers are more concerned about that than the idea of dying.
Nurse:	Bill, it sounds as if, even now, you are more concerned about the effects of this on your wife and others than on yourself.
Bill:	Well, I guess I always have tried to consider others.
Analysis:	Reinforcing Bill's strength and his concern for others which may provide sufficient meaning for him to deal with this crisis.
Nurse:	I think your wife doesn't know quite how to cope with this whole situation.
Bill:	Yes, she has always relied on me to get through the tough times.
Analysis:	Shifting to needs of wife in order to determine ego strength and coping energy Bill can presently tap.
Nurse:	Bill, you are an amazing man in the way you are coping with this illness and yet being so concerned about others.
Bill:	Well, I just wish I could make it easier for her.
Analysis:	Nurse reinforces Bill's self-concept while recognizing his present need for denial of the full impact of his condition.
Nurse:	Can the two of you talk about things you can do to make it a little easier for each other?

(continued)

214 Caring for the Psychogeriatric Client

TABLE 6.6 (continued)

Bill:	No, I've been trying to protect her.
Nurse:	I can understand your desire to do that but not knowing what to do or say is pretty tough. Can the three of us talk together now?
Bill:	O.K.
Analysis:	Before leaving the situation the nurse must be concerned about developing some reciprocal supports for each of the distressed persons. Too often, each spouse lives in silent misery in a misguided attempt to protect the other.

- Conflicting myths: Life is fair/life is controllable; one is teleologic, the other anthropomorphic. Control in the first is external and in the second it is internal.
- The nurse concentrated energy in the dialectic process of modifying the client's expectation of diametrically opposed expectations.
- The individual seemed best able to cope by maintaining a sense of his internal control. While recognizing that some things were beyond his control, he was able to regain his sense of efficacy.
- His anchor at this time was in the belief that his actions would affect others in negative or positive ways, thus that control had both internal and external aspects.

Summary of Nursing Care Plan   The following extrapolates from the sample case above and summarizes general nursing care principles for patients at risk of suicide.

Assessment

- Client is at high risk of suicide.
- Client is depressed.
- Client has a lingering illness with the expectation of death.
- Client initially expresses feelings of helplessness.
- Client is experiencing decreased self-regard.
- Client is not judged lethal at this time.

Goals of Intervention with Suicidal Elder

- Determine suicide potential.
- Protect the individual from suicide if necessary.
- Strengthen existing support systems.

- Enhance self-esteem and sense of control.
- Restore meaning by modification of conflicting myths.

Outcome Criteria

- Does client demonstrate a more positive affect?
- Does client have more eye contact?
- Does client move about in a more decisive way?
- Does client leave bed or bedroom?
- Does client appear more comfortable or relaxed?
- Does client make effort to include his wife?

Evaluation of Progress Toward Goals

- Client is ambivalent about his situation.
- Client is experiencing some denial.
- Client maintains a strong sense of self.
- Client is not immediately suicidal.
- Client has a functional support system.
- Client will put his wife's needs prior to his own.
- Client is beginning to restore his sense of meaning.

DSM III-R Classification

- *Mood Congruent Depressive Episode Related to Life Circumstance Problem Associated with Physical Condition* (This demonstrates with some clarity the difficulty of applying DSM III-R categories realistically to many of the emotional disorders of aging. The most common disorders are the result of intertwined biopsychosocial assaults.)

Psychiatric Nursing Diagnosis

- *Alterations in thought content with suicidal ideation related to temporarily altered ability to constructively manage stress of confrontation with terminal illness.*

Secondary Diagnosis

- Alterations in self-care related to decreased interest and loss of confidence in body.
- Impaired emotional experience of distress/anguish related to internal conflicts and spiritual distress regarding beliefs.

- Impaired family role related to feelings of helplessness and dependence.
- Alterations in self concept: impaired personal identity related to powerlessness over impending illness and death.
- Impaired function of defenses related to turning against self.
- Alterations in sleep pattern related to insomnia as a result of emotional stress.
- Deficit in bowel elimination due to inactivity and insufficient intake.
- Alterations in nutrition: anorexia related to emotional stress.
- Impaired range of emotional focus related to premature grief.

Interventions

- Discussion of suicidal thoughts.
- Encourage verbalization of feelings.
- Protect from harming self.
- Encourage decision making.
- Treat with dignity and respect.
- Assist to resolve conflicting values and expectations.
- Restore or reinforce interpersonal relations.
- Support biologic functions.

Life-Review and Suicide

The most characteristically traditional psychotherapeutic intervention with aged persons is assisting with "life-review"—a term coined by Butler (1963). In brief, the process can be equated with that of psychoanalysis wherein the individual harbors conflicting feelings or remorse regarding certain remote events that remain unresolved or inadequately understood. The life-review process seems to occur spontaneously when an aged individual experiences a disruptive event that triggers the resurgence of unresolved and painful memories (see Chapter 4). A nonjudgmental and warm approach by the caregiver encourages resolution. The goal is to assist the individual to accept his or her life course with a sense of peace, or at least to reduce harsh self-judgment. To further clarify life-review, an example is presented below.

J. was admitted to a mental health center after being found extremely intoxicated in a public telephone booth. He was angry and belligerent and seemed unable to remember how he had come to be hospitalized. A health history determined that he was 78 years old with no major health problems. His wife had died of cancer nine months previously and he had no other significant relationships.

The immediate caregiving priority was to hydrate him and provide good nourishment as it seemed he had neglected himself recently. A particularly caring atmosphere was needed to partially compensate for the deficit he experienced upon the demise of his wife, as well.

One week after admission J. was restored physically but his affectual tone of sadness predominated. The psychiatric nursing diagnosis concluded that J. experienced *aggressive/violence toward self, which was expressed in substance abuse and possible suicidal thoughts related to impaired grieving.*

Nurse B. spent time with him each day encouraging him to express his thoughts and grief. He spoke of how he missed his wife. He also spoke of the guilt he felt over brief sexual escapades during their marriage and that he had felt unable to express his tender feelings toward his wife. He believed his wife to be an extraordinarily "good" woman and blamed himself relentlessly for his unfaithfulness and lack of appreciation for his wife while she lived. He regretted that he could not now ask forgiveness and express how intensely he loved her. Obviously, this man could be considered in the midst of a life-review and seeking restitution, forgiveness, and release. The nurse employed the following methods of assisting him:

- Role playing; in which she acted as his wife and encouraged him to express everything he would like to have said to her.
- Reminiscing about all the pleasant events he could remember about his marriage.
- Talking about his wife, describing her attributes and her faults.
- Guiding him through a fantasy of what he would like his life with her to have been.
- Reassuring him that his grief process was proceeding and that his thoughts were not abnormal.
- Encouraging him to write a letter to his wife expressing all that he would like to have said before she died.
- Discussing thoughts of suicide that he might have.
- Helping him construct a list of all persons he knew that might provide social outlets for him.
- Staying with him while he initiated phone contact with an old friend.
- Involving him in a day care program prior to discharge.

Persons like J. have often isolated themselves and have lost the desire to interact. Day care programs and senior centers provide myriad services to meet multiple needs and provide contact with other seniors. J. undoubtedly would resist attending and would need to be accompanied the first time by Nurse B., with whom he had begun to establish human contact. It would be most helpful if he could participate in a way that demonstrated some of his abilities and talents. In addition, he might be guided to a grief support group. Sloan (1978) likens the psychiatric care of an aged person to wartime psychiatry. The goal is to keep the patient mobile, out of the hospital, and involved with activities and relationships.

PARANOIA

Paranoia is a frequent accompaniment of the assaults and cognitive changes of old age. In middle and late life, when present, it is most often a chronic state of mind with few periods of exacerbation or remission. The determination of the presence of paranoia versus the reality of suspicion based upon sound reasons presents a significant problem, however. Paranoia is unfounded fear and suspicion which may be specific to certain persons and situations or more generalized. It often accompanies delirium, dementias, and social isolation. Other conditions that may result in paranoia include: hypoglycemia; alcohol withdrawal; drugs, such as cortisone, methyltestosterone, anticholinergics, barbiturates, L-dopa, and imipramine; and uremia. Less severe and disabling paranoia is often observed following relocation, severe stress, and in those with impaired hearing. Also, I have frequently observed the emergence of paranoid feelings due to hypoxia that subside when the oxygen deficit is compensated. Paranoia disorders are further illustrated in the list below. Characteristics were summarized from the DSM III-R (1987).

PARANOID DISORDERS

Onset: Middle or late life
         Chronic with few periods of exacerbation or remission
         Acute (limited to 6 months) unusual in late life

Predisposing Factors:
         Immigration/relocation
         Impaired hearing
         Severe stress

Causes Common to Aged
         Organic dementias
         Delirium
         Hypoglycemia
         Alcohol abuse/withdrawal psychoses
         Cortisone/methyltestosterone
         Anticholinergic agents
         Barbiturates/imipramine
         L-dopa
         Isolation

Projective mechanisms to cope with ageism
Uremia

Responses
Suspicion often based on core of truth
Internalized rejection
Realistic wariness
Expectation of being explioted or harmed
Guarded

Interventions
Reduce anxiety
Consistency in expectations
Focus attention on successes
Enhance coping
Increase self-esteem
Establish reliable interpersonal resource

Suspicion, on the other hand, is less disabling, carries less fear with it, and may be exhibited in extreme caution and compulsive behaviors that maintain a sense of control and predictability. Two examples show that there is often good reason for suspicion that may be judged as paranoia.

Walt was annoyed because the doctor visting him in the nursing home never really stopped to listen to him. The "shirt-tail" visits, as Walt called them, were cursory at best. He explained that he never had time to grab his shirt-tail before the doctor was gone. His solution was to put a tape recorder in his room and attempt to tape the doctor's visit to provide evidence of his neglect. The doctor discovered the tape recorder and referred Walt to a psychiatrist for assessment of his "paranoia." A nurse who was well aware of the whole scenario acted as advocate for Walt and nothing came of the event. Lacking the nurse's intervention, it could readily have resulted in a diagnosis of paranoia and all the attendant medications and lack of confidence in the patient's judgment.

In another instance, a physician in an emergency room in New York City said, "When anyone brings an aged person in saying he/she is paranoid, I immediately ask myself, Who wants her apartment?"

Realistic wariness and caution are self-sustaining and are a strength rather than a problem. As one psychiatrist put it succinctly, "Anyone who is not suspicious is really crazy!" This seems to be particularly true of the aged who are so often taken advantage of by family, friends, and our social priority system.

Certain suggestions that may prove useful in dealing with suspiciousness and paranoia are provided in the list below.

INTERVENTIONS FOR PARANOIA AND SUSPICIOUSNESS

Check out the reality of the fears and suspicions.
Reduce anxiety by giving information prior to instituting
any action.
Establish consistent expectations.
Enhance daily coping skills.
Focus patient attention on small gains and successes.
Increase self-esteem through providing opportunities for
decision making.
Establish a reliable relationship with the patient.
Avoid engaging in competitive activities.
Assist client to develop a daily schedule and follow it.

Brink (1984) reported an attempt to construct a Late Life Paranoia
Scale (LLPS) that could be answered by geriatric clients and would be
predictive of paranoid thought processes. It was found to be unreli-
able as the development of paranoid thoughts in old age was too
diverse and situationally dependent to be surveyed with consistency.
Related to this finding are those earlier studies of Colby (1977) and
Sands (1983) that demonstrated paranoia as a defense against shame
and assaults to self-esteem precipitated by actual life events. For
nurses, the most important of their findings are that the intensity of
paranoia abates as self-esteem rises.

Some theorists speculate that demented persons are more likely to
interpret the environment as threatening and thus feel suspicious and
develop paranoia. Brink et al. (1985) failed to demonstrate any correlation between paranoia and dementia when using a Stimulus Recognition test (SRT). While these reports were not conclusive in any
respect, they provide new insights that nurses may indeed pursue as
items of clinical research.

CONCLUSION

This chapter has addressed psychogeriatric disorders of an acute
nature that often precipitate hospitalization. However, because the
manic side of mood disorders are less frequently seen than depressions in later life, they were not dealt with here. Adjustment and sleep
disorders were included in Chapters 4 and 5 and are not usual causes
for acute-care hospitalizations. Anxiety disorders may precipitate hospitalization but are diffuse in their origins and thus have not claimed a

specific category in this chapter. Gender and sexual disorders are often dealt with, if at all, as a medical problem. Nonetheless, caregivers need to give more attention to these problems in psychiatric care. In addition, personality disorders are so often a matter of interpretation by the beholder that they have also been excluded here. Still, the most pertinent problems have been addressed so as to assist in their management in the psychogeriatric setting. Many of the suggestions offered will also be useful in long-term care settings and community care modes.

7

Families and Caregiving

Whether or not they are willing or have the personal and economic resources, family and other primary caregivers bear the burden of caring for elders. As a result, an enormous number of descriptive studies of family caregivers and their needs have appeared during the past several years, although only parsimonious real assistance has been provided. In the decade of the 1990s, however, caring for elders will be a high priority among policy makers and the population in general as we individually and collectively are more frequently confronted with the enormity of need for supportive care. Understanding this need, industries, such as IBM, are even now providing resources through employee assistance programs to those employees who find their work affected by the needs and demands of elder relatives.

Because they so often fall within health care categories that are not reimbursable, the psychologic needs of elders and their caregivers require particular attention. This chapter provides information related to recent studies and suggestions for caring for elders and their family caregivers. In this respect, the family, which is still the matrix of our society, must be reinforced, respected, and strengthened.

222

FAMILY CAREGIVERS

Caregiver is a word generally used to describe someone who provides informal, unpaid care to an elder person who requires assistance with daily routines and to meet personal needs. Although it is often thought otherwise, family caregivers provide from 70 to 80% of all care given to elders. As such, professional and paraprofessional caregivers often find that the *family* is as much the client as the elder who has the identified problem and is the "ticket bearer" in the health care system. Because the professional caregivers' role is to provide support, assistance, and education to the family as the most natural and effective way of helping elders, I have included extensive information about families and their needs and propensities.

CAREGIVING IN THE HOME

As hospital costs are higher, reimbursement lower, and rapid discharge to home or nursing home more usual than not, home health care has become increasingly important as the locus of care delivery. Often, family who are poorly prepared to do so shoulder the major burden of care and rehabilitation. The professional caregiver's task is to assist them in finding the most appropriate and economic benefits and to strengthen their resolve in pursuing them. Home health care will provide services that include: nursing, physical therapy, speech and hearing therapy, occupational therapy, nutritional counseling, social services, laboratory services, dental care, transportation, supplies and equipment. However, patient need must be verified and a physician's order for home health care is required. Home health agencies can be located through local hospitals, Area Agencies on Aging, local or county public health departments, and the Yellow Pages of the telephone directory. Medicare coverage for services is limited to skilled care and is not usually available for maintenance of supportive services or for the individual with chronic long-term illness. Specific services not covered by Medicare include: full-time nursing care, most drugs, meals, homemaker or chore services, and custodial or personal services.

Some of the services that are available at minimal or no cost to families and have markedly improved their caregiving abilities include: day care programs, telephone reassurance, friendly visitors, hospice, Meals-on-Wheels, respite care, and transportation programs. Family and friends can also reduce the cost of home care assistants by assisting with personal hygiene, laundry, changing linens, house cleaning, preparing meals, grocery shopping, assisting person to ambulate, and giving medications.

If problems occur with the quality or reliability of home care services provided by an agency, the local Consumer Affairs Office should be notified. Consumers should know that there is evidence of inadequate staff training, poor supervision, poor care, and abuses attributed to some home health agencies, as well as significant variations in cost of services. To ensure quality, appropriate cost, and reliability, the American Association of Retired Persons (AARP) suggests investigating the following items listed below before selecting an agency.

CHECKLIST FOR SELECTING AND EVALUATING
HOME HEALTH AGENCY

Selection.
Wide range of services available.
Available hours and days of week when needed.
Number of qualified supervisors.
Availability of physician consultation.
Certification and accreditation verifiable.
Current operating license.
Clear criteria for eligibility.
Evaluation of service provided.
Patient (family) can contact staff or physician.
Physician visits patient when necessary.
Supervisor visits patient periodically.
Patient informed of care plan and progress.
Periodic reassessment of care plan is made.
Services expected are received.
Questions and concerns are answered.
Scheduled visits are kept.

Home Care of Emotionally Disturbed Elders

Home care, either after acute-care hospitalization, or to manage problems in the home to prevent the need for hospitalization, has become a predominant mode of patient management. Many health maintenance organizations (HMOs) are particularly well prepared to provide a continuum of services to reduce the need for acute hospital care. Few HMOs, however, provide mental health services. The following case study, therefore, exemplifies the complexity of medical and psychosocial issues impinging on care and the knowledge needed by home care providers.

At present, the most common approach to caring for the mentally disturbed elder in the home is to rely on medication; supportive groups and educational programs for family members; and respite care and day care on a fee-for-service basis to provide intermittent relief to overburdened family members.

Case Study for Analysis and Development of Home Care Plan   Myrna was an 80-year-old white female of German heritage who lived in a double level tract home in a suburb of San Francisco. She resided there with her brother, 20 years her junior and never married. Myrna's husband had been a cruise ship steward prior to his death two years ago. Myrna's husband was rarely in port and, therefore, her brother, Herb, served as companion and Myrna treated him as she would a son. Myrna had no children. She was rather "well fixed" financially but due to childhood deprivation was very frugal. Herb had worked in a lumber yard since his retirement from the U.S. Navy. Myrna and Herb rarely visited anyone except for the young family next door to whom they served as surrogate grandparents. Occasionally, the close neighbors would hear them in heated argument over Herb's drinking, Myrna's smoking, and the ladies of Herb's acquaintance of whom Myrna did not approve. Relatives would visit rarely; basically Myrna and Herb were quite reclusive.

Myrna's motivation in life seemed to come from her need to "keep up appearances." Like many of her generation, she was greatly concerned about what others thought of her. She led a very circumspect life and while she claimed to have no religious leanings she always attended church when the children next door invited her to their holiday programs.

Myrna's youth had been hard. Born on a farm in Missouri, the eldest of 12 children, she had hardly known a carefree moment in childhood. She still spoke of her mother and father with some bitterness. Apparently, her father drank and the mother spent most of her days in exhausted depression, leaving the care of the family to Myrna. When she was 16 years old, Myrna left home and went to work as a waitress in Chicago. She often spoke of how she finally worked her way into the Palmer House in Chicago and what a coup that was for her. She met and married Arthur while there and migrated to the West Coast where he began his career as a steward. Myrna thought the accessibility of drugs in the Orient was one of the attractions of the career Arthur chose. In any case, he developed a strong dependence on various kinds of illegal drugs. Myrna spent most of her working life as a waitress in such places as the St. Francis and Palace Hotels. She enjoyed her work and keeping a "well-appointed" home.

Myrna's health history is vague in regard to childhood illnesses. It is assumed that within a large family of her generation she must have experienced most of the known childhood illnesses. She had never had surgery or physically traumatic events and had always been lithe and small. Her young adulthood was during the time of prohibition and bathtub gin and she had indulged in most of the antics of that era. Other than heavy drinking in her youth and moderate smoking most of her life, Myrna led a healthy life style. She was never a faddist and consumed a broad variety of foods. She had little physical exercise and did not seem to desire any.

While Myrna had stopped school at fifth grade to care for small children in the home, she was bright and had a large library which she enjoyed. She especially loved poetry and history. She had never attempted to obtain more formal education.

Myrna's health problems began a year after her husband died. She began to have difficulty breathing and after a thorough workup she was diagnosed by her Kaiser physician as having incipient cataracts, late onset diabetes, and emphysema. Having felt healthy all of her life, Myrna was quite shaken by these diagnoses. Being the type of person she was, there was never any problem in her compliance with whatever the physician prescribed, yet her condition steadily deteriorated over the year. At this time, she began experiencing periods of confusion, disorientation, and extreme suspicion of others. To help her, Herb hired several maids for the home but Myrna always fired them within a day or two after accusing them of stealing from her. In addition, Herb couldn't sleep because Myrna wandered at night and called out threats to anyone she thought may have mistreated her. Herb called Kaiser (HMO) for assistance as he felt Myrna needed hospitalization. A home health nurse was sent out to assess the situation.

Prioritizing Needs through Use of Diagnoses   To develop a home care plan for Myrna, one must prioritize needs and problems. The Taxonomy of Psychiatric Nursing Diagnoses (PND) is a useful approach in her case (Psychiatric Nursing Phenomona Task Force, 1986).

Biologic responses.
Social/behavioral responses.
Emotional responses.
Defensive responses.
Perceptual responses.

When one applies this organizational hierarchy to the resolution of the most immediate problems, less pressing problems are often partially ameliorated as well.

In Myrna's case, the home health nurse judged problems and needs to be as follows:

- Biologic: Inadequate oxygenation, nutritional/metabolic alterations, sensory deficits, possible alcohol related impairment.

  Needs: Medication monitoring, evaluation of oxygenation, nutritional evaluation and education, portable oxygen availability, evaluation for cataract surgery.

- Social/behavioral: Sleep disturbances, agitation, wandering, verbal abusiveness, diversional activity deficits, role loss/conflict.

Needs: Daytime activity (possibly Talking Books, Day Care Center, contact with minister of church), sitter at night until sleep pattern stabilized.

• Emotional: Mood disturbance (depression, irritability, mistrust), displaced anger, possible impaired grief process.

Needs: Ventilation of feelings, stress reduction techniques.

• Defensive: Inappropriate defenses, displacement, and projection exhibited in suspiciousness.

Needs: Consistent and direct feedback as well as clear explanations of expectations.

• Perceptual: Impaired judgment, impaired sensory processing, impaired personal identity, social identity, and self-esteem.

Needs: Life-history review, identification of strengths.

Application of Psychiatric Nursing Diagnoses to Myrna's Case

Alterations in metabolic function related to diabetes.
Possible alterations in sensory function related to cataracts.
Alterations in oxygenation (dyspnea) related to emphysema.
Alterations in impulse control related to delusions: verbally abusive and potentially assaultive.
Alterations in role performance related to failing health: potential dependence.
Impaired social role related to social isolation and suspicion.
Alterations in sleep arousal related to metabolic disturbances and hypoxia.
Excess of dominant emotions: grief, anger, anxiety, fear, and help-lessness related to lack of empathetic support persons and loss of health and roles.
Excess defensiveness demonstrated in projection of fears related to feelings of helplessness.
Impaired judgment and thought processes related to hypoxia and lack of personal feedback.
Potential disorientation.
Impaired social identity related to isolation.

Appropriate DSM III-R Diagnoses in this Case

Non-substance-induced delusional syndrome due to metabolic imbalances.

Sleep/arousal disorders due to chronic obstructive pulmonary disease (COPD).
Generalized anxiety due to failing health.
Passive/aggressive personality disorder due to repressed anger.

The home health nurse must be astute to address psychosocial needs and simultaneously provide care for physical needs. In this case, there will be periodic visits to evaluate maintenance in the home situation. It is economically and psychologically advantageous for Myrna to remain in the home as long as possible. As Herb is her major support, he will need respite and attention to his needs.

In a health agency without the provision of comprehensive home services and only Medicare reimbursement for home health care, caregivers would expect, just as Herb did, rapid deterioration and placement in an institution.

Evaluation

Evaluation of success or progress in meeting mutually defined goals with aged persons must be ongoing and continually modified to reflect changes in self-esteem, coping capacity, support network, and physical status.

Family Caregivers and their Stressors

Lehr (1987) found that unmarried middle-aged daughters were the most likely caregivers for aged parents. In addition, those with interests, work, or activities outside the home were most likely to cope effectively with caregiving demands. Lehr also found that intergenerational relationships during the earlier years had a marked effect on the perceived stress in the present caretaking role.

Borden, Frankel & Gierl (1987) correlated psychological well-being in the caregiver role with high levels of social support and ability to use a broad range of coping skills. These are important considerations for health care personnel who may be used as consultants or support persons to family caregivers.

Caring for an elderly family member can disturb family routines, reactivate unresolved relationship issues, stimulate regressive behavior in various family members, and threaten the well-being of each family member. Invisible loyalties in family relationships and certain family traditions may influence patterns of caregiving, as well. The requirements of caregiving require role changes that provoke development of new coping techniques: social, economic, and psychodynamic. If understanding and support are available, the challenge can be growth promoting.

Toward that end, a mutually constructed, written assessment of a family's needs and coping capacities can be comprehensive and specific enough to become a document of family strengths in times of stress. Foci to be included are: sources of stress, particular coping methods, resources that are used or can be used, and the rewards and problems of caregiving. While staff are cognizant of the need for written care plans and evaluation of patient progress, this may not be shared with or given to the family. Inclusion in the development of a nursing care plan and periodic evaluation may help the family assess their effectiveness even in the face of patient decline.

In addition, it is important that family members know the factors that emerge as indices of coping in the caregiving role, including: perceived well-being, perceived social support, promotion of functional ability of the care-receiver, and positive relationship to care-receiver.

In terms of the caregivers' intrapsychic world and interpersonal network, however, much less is known. In fact, strengths and weaknesses of the caregiver should be more carefully investigated in future research on associated distress.

For example, planning and providing psychological, supportive, and therapeutic services for caregivers may be equally or more important than more concrete services, such as day care or respite.

In this vein, Matthiesen (1987) studied adult daughters' relationship with their institutionalized mothers, concentrating on the daughters' personal and emotional lives. In exploring the need for daughters to adapt to their mothers' institutionalization, it was apparent that a major personal transition was experienced in which new social and psychological dimensions of their nature emerged. Redefining one's role in this sense also involved stages of disorganization, flux, and resolution. Depicting such stages can be useful in understanding and supporting daughters as well as other family members through the difficult adjustment they face. Though not addressed by this study, it is likely that daughters may also be dealing with anticipation of their own aging experience and potential for similar placement.

Families of Alzheimer's Victims

Alzheimer's disease is a progressive, relentless, and deteriorating disorder of mind with no known specific cause or effective treatment. While many studies have provided precise descriptions of brain tissue changes and enzyme deficiencies, the problem facing families is of another sort: It occurs in the daily management of an individual who is essentially a stranger. Personality, lifestyle, habits, and feelings are often unrecognizable as that of the loved one. To add to the difficulty, with the erosion of personal judgment objectionable personality bents that had not been expressed become apparent.

Early in the course of the disease, almost imperceptible changes in the individual's ability to function may result in daily irritations in family life that cause distress and disgust. By the time the disease is diagnosable, these may have already built a barrier in the relationships with loved ones. Unpaid bills, carelessness with grooming and eating, repetitious questions, and forgetfulness have already eroded the responsiveness and caring concern of those in close contact. To compensate, family and friends may unwittingly delay confrontation with the real problem as they attribute these changes to "old age" or simple thoughtlessness. Commonly, frustration, anger, and resentment are already manifest, however, before the enormity of the problem is known or confronted. In addition, facing the problem involves all the stages of grief with which caregivers are familiar: denial, anger, bargaining, working through, and acceptance. Unfortunately, when grief over the lost personality of the loved one is complete, the shell of the individual may remain to cause daily problems for many years. As a result, the family becomes exhausted, drained, and emotionally devastated. McNulty and Dann (1984, pp. 34–38) share some of the comments of family members that provide insight into their feelings regarding a member with Alzheimer's disease.

It is a funeral that never ends.

I feel that I am witnessing the prolonged, living death of a person who was once one thing and who now is nothing. And in witnessing her living death, I end up being a weekly mourner. I sometimes resent that I can't go to church without crying.

There was a sort of gleeful maliciousness in some of my reactions to her, particularly in terms of my being more competent than she was.

Of course everytime I forget something . . . I have visions of myself in my mother's condition.

And there are other families who somehow manage by accepting the challenge and giving it meaning:

I have many friends and interests and these I am able to do at home. In fact, wild parties have been known to go on with my husband sleeping peacefully in his chair in the midst of all the fun and games, so it is not all gloom and doom. I shall keep him at home unless I have to give up at some time, but I feel I have got so far that it will have to be really drastic for me to stop. I would not have missed this experience. It would be nice if he could speak, but holding hands and being silent can also pass on a lot."

In a 1983 speech, Nancy Mace of the Johns Hopkins Alzheimer's research team and co-author of *The 36-Hour Day* (1981), said:

> Clearly, for some patients, some of the time, having dementia is not synonymous with suffering but these success stories are rare. They are far outnumbered by stories of patient suffering and family suffering.

To further illustrate this problem, see Figure 7.1 for needs of family members caring for elders with senile dementia of the Alzheimer's type. The need for family respite services has been widely discussed but little has been done to provide sufficient assistance. Adult day care centers that care for the impaired elder have provided

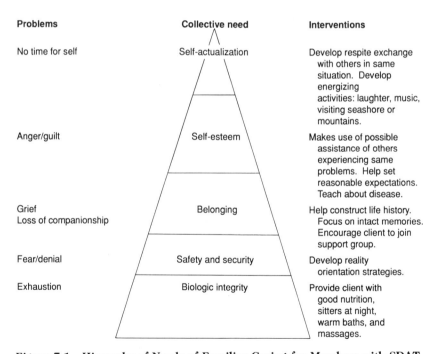

Figure 7.1   Hierarchy of Needs of Families Caring for Members with SDAT.

Source: From P. Ebersole & P. Hess. (1985). *Toward Healthy Aging: Human Needs and Nursing Response,* 2nd Ed. St. Louis; C. V. Mosby.

Caring for the Psychogeriatric Client

the most effective service but are often cost prohibitive to the family or the hours may be so limited as to make it impractical for working spouses to enroll their elder member. In response to these needs, the Robert Wood Johnson Foundation, in conjunction with the Alzheimer's Disease and Related Disorders Association and the Administration on Aging, has developed a national Dementia Care and Respite Services Program that will provide grants in the range of $250,000 to $300,000 over a four-year period (from 1988 to 1992) to as many as 25 adult day centers across the United States. The potential success of this effort will have great significance in the lives of the burdened middle generation as well as providing a viable alternative model to premature institutionalization of some vulnerable elders.

In-home respite care remains the most frequently used caregiving mode. It involves giving the primary caregiver some time out of the house, a few hours, a day, a week, or more. The patient remains in familiar surroundings and the caregiver retains control over all decisions related to patient care. Sources of respite care may be formal, informal, paid, or unpaid. Friends and family, church members, members of organized cooperatives who exchange respite services, and paid companion/homemakers are some sources of in-home respite care. If the patient's condition warrants, a nurse's aide, vocational nurse, or registered nurse may be necessary. For an individual with dementia, changes of environment may exacerbate problems. In-home respite care, therefore, is most desirable for such an individual when that is feasible.

Out-of-home respite care may be obtained in day care centers, institutions with beds allocated for respite service, foster care, or board and care. In some cases, very creative solutions have been devised. For example, families rotate the elder to the various family member's homes for certain periods. In Boise, Idaho, a program was instituted by the Mountain States Health Corporation and funded by the Fred Meyer Foundation to match patients with individuals in the community who were willing to provide residential day care for one or two persons. The personal attention and individualized care in those situations seemed beneficial.

Schwartz (1987) notes that the vast majority of elders with mild to moderate degrees of impairment live at home and are treated by physicians on an outpatient basis. To assess subtle changes in patient status, the physician will need an alliance with the family in which their knowledge of the patient is respected and carefully considered. Significant others are an excellent source of information concerning relevant changes in social functioning, activities of daily living, memory functioning, and personal care and grooming. Therefore, it is incumbent upon physicians and family members to cooperate as completely as possible to ensure quality of care for the impaired elder.

Brody (1985) has consistently demonstrated the commitment and responsible behaviors of most families. In addition, Brody has identified the following as roles commonly assumed by family members. Family members:

- Act as decisionmakers for the impaired.
- Act as principal sources of emotional support.
- Act as socializing agents for the impaired.
- Mobilize and coordinate services.
- Offer financial support and money management.
- Act as mediators and advocates with "formal" support systems.
- Provide personal care and medically related care (80–90%).
- Provide instrumental services (shopping, home maintenance, and transportation).
- Share homes and provide living space.

The family role is so central to survival and quality of life for frail elders (Harel & Noelker, 1978) that caregivers must consider the total family as the client when planning for the impaired elder. Assessment of the family's caregiving capacity and availability of resources must be coupled with assessment of the needs of the elderly member.

Elder Abuse by Caregivers

Studies of abuse victims indicate that the social deterioration and functional incapacity inherent in certain disorders most often incite abuse from caregivers or abusive actions from the aged individual. For example, during the admission of his wife to a mental health unit, I overheard one aged man state that he had to "spank" her to help her behave.

Abuse may occur in response to the following conditions:

Organic delusional syndrome.
Primary degenerative dementia.
Organic hallucinosis.
Dementia associated with alcoholism.
Dependent personality disorders.
Passive/aggressive disorders.
Obsessive/compulsive disorders.
Generalized anxiety disorders.

In stating a nursing diagnosis, it is always essential to focus on the actual exhibited behavior rather than the psychiatric diagnosis. The nursing diagnosis must also be qualified in terms of possibility, probability, potentiality, and actual presence; for example, potential abuse related to constant repetitious babbling of patient as a result of primary degenerative dementia of the late stage. Such detailed statements make resolution much easier to define. For instance, the constancy of apparently meaningless behavior exhibited by a patient is extremely frustrating for the caregiver unless there are periods of relief or the behavior can be controlled. Given the diagnosis of late stage dementia, it is also improbable the patient can control this behavior. A search of the literature, however, would reveal that Zachow (1984) found several interventions useful in relating to one elderly lady demonstrating similar behavior (see Chapter 4). Spaced multisensorial approaches to the patient, touch, one-to-one attention in comfortable surroundings, and Baroque music were found to result in some meaningful communication from the patient. Planning to institute some of these activities would constitute an initial intervention. Followup, encouragement, and timing would constitute another important intervention. Evaluation and modification of the plan would rely upon the caregiver's assessment of improvement in regard to the offensive behavior. If it is found that the interventions based on Zachow's limited strategies are not effective with this particular elderly person, it must be assumed that inherent individual differences have limited the applicability of those strategies.

However, if the nurse determines that the actual client in this case is a family or a family caregiver, then prevention of abuse becomes the desired long-term goal and changing offensive behavior to relieve stress on the caregiver becomes the desired short-term goal. The nurse would then revise the plan and attempt to assist the family caregiver to construct possibilities of respite, to develop workable stress reduction strategies, and to alert him or her to sources of help when the situation begins to feel intolerable. Reduction of stressors in other areas of the caregiver's lifestyle may be sufficient to maintain constructive coping behaviors. In other words, sometimes the approach to problem solving must be indirect and the client may be one or more persons, a family, neighborhood, or even an entire community. For additional, in-depth information and case studies regarding elder abuse, I recommend Quinn and Tomita's (1987) Elder Abuse and Neglect.

LONG-DISTANCE CAREGIVING

Long-distance caregiving is more frequent and more devastating than one might expect. In a mobile society, children of the impaired or disabled elder may be geographically removed but emotionally and financially heavily involved in the care of their loved one. Often, the inclination is to relocate the elder and this is done precipitously without considering the roots and needs of the elder or the ramifications for the family. There are some specific ways to make the most of a long-distance and caring relationship. As you work with families, some of these may be discussed.

First, family members must try to banish feelings of guilt. The elder may much prefer maintaining the quality of the relationship at a distance rather than eroding it through becoming a "necessary burden." Second, visits should be scheduled in advance and allow enough time for family members to observe the realities of daily life for the elder. What services may be really needed and how family members can assist in obtaining them while visiting are significant concerns. Third, suggest family members and the elder talk honestly about feelings and perceptions of the situation. Family members should be cautioned to listen carefully to the elder's viewpoints. They may be quite divergent. Fourth, discuss with family members the development of a contingency plan in the event more assistance becomes necessary. Plans made in haste during an emergency situation may not be well thought out. Fifth, and last, ask family members to identify the informal network already in existence for the elder and reinforce it where possible. Contact and reaffirm the importance of these individuals periodically after the return home.

A network of services are beginning to emerge to assist geographically distant family members in ensuring that an elder relative will be taken care of. In many cases, a "case manager" approach is being used in which the individual calls a care coordinating entrepreneurial resource broker. Some nurses and social workers have seen the need and are developing this type of service (see resource in Appendix F). Because this service is not presently covered by private insurance or public agencies of any kind, it is only available to those who are able to pay.

FAMILIES AND INSTITUTIONALIZATION

Assisting a family to make wise decisions regarding long-term care may be one of the most important tasks of health care professionals. Often, long-term care is equated with nursing homes when in reality there are other options suitable for certain persons. When round-the-clock care is needed, then a nursing home may be the most suitable. If assistance is needed with meals and personal care, an individual may best be served by a residential care home, board and care home, congregate housing, or a retirement community. Often, particular decisions must be made based on cost. It is important the family and elder be well informed about exact costs, services, and any assistance for which they are qualified. It is equally important to consider the elements of lifestyle most cherished by the elder and endeavor to find a situation in which they are most likely to be maintained. To aid in this search for relevant information, the AARP has prepared a packet of *Resources for Caregivers*, available from the national office (see appendices for address, the checklist of concerns/resources, and bibliography of useful publications.)

Persons at greatest risk of requiring nursing home care are very elderly ladies with dementia who are poor and without available family who are capable and willing to provide care. Many elderly men in similar straits may be found within the Veterans Administration Hospital system. However, nearly 15% of elderly in institutions have a spouse and about half have adult children. The more living children one has, the less likely one will require a nursing home. Yet the need for long-term care at some time during late life is projected for up to 40% of elders (HCFA, 1982). Therefore, the often cited statistic that only 5% of the elderly are in nursing homes is misleading if not understood as only cross-sectional data. The discharge rate from nursing homes must also be examined critically as two-thirds of the time the patient is merely discharged to another facility or hospital rather than to home.

These statistics are presented to underscore the fact that families, with few exceptions, will be compelled to deal with the long-term care of at least one of their elder members. They must also anticipate the possibility of movement between long-term care facilities, acute-care hospitals, and community agencies. All of this, of course, is emotionally taxing to the family and the elder.

Mary, for example, had lived in one nursing home for six years and felt quite secure in that environment. Following a fall she was transferred to acute care and when stabilized was transferred to another nursing home as her bed in the previous facility was no longer available. Mary became extremely disorganized and disoriented in the new setting. She simply did not have the psychic energy at that time to adapt to a new environment and new demands. Her family misunderstood her deterioration in cognitive function and assumed she was developing "Alzheimer's disease." It was threatening to them and they began to distance themselves when she needed them most. Lacking adequate psychosocial support and family understanding, Mary did retreat farther from reality and the family's fears became a self-fulfilled prophecy.

Tragically, greater awareness by family members could have helped to prevent Mary's deterioration. For example, a family member may have been able to provide the continuity so desperately needed by

Mary merely by accompanying her and providing support in each of her transfers. In addition, the administration of the first nursing home might have offered Mary's family the option of paying to hold the bed open for Mary's return, if that was deemed desirable.

What, then should families do to promote mental health of members who are nursing home residents? There are many "shoulds" reflecting the values, bias, economic considerations, and political ideology of the proponent. Presently, it is popular to shift toward more, rather than less, family responsibility for elders. Indeed, some states tried to implement a federal law passed in 1983 to force families to pay for the institutional care of aged parents. The implication, of course, is clear: it assumes that families must be legally required to care for their members.

Despite the frequency with which it occurs families are rarely psychologically prepared for the elder individual's need for institutionalization. The shock felt by each family member when institutionalization becomes a necessity can be severe enough to precipitate a crisis. As the conflict between relief and sorrow complicates the adjustment process, feelings of guilt and shame may be aroused as well. As a result, relationship problems will often be exacerbated, latent sibling rivalries will appear, and anxieties about aging and death can no longer be ignored. The following case study exemplifies such problems.

It became apparent that Ella was unable to manage alone in her home after her husband's death. She made a marginal adjustment at first but in her depressed state she neglected nutrition, exercise, and rest. She also took numerous medications from the well-stocked "pharmacy" with which she had been amply supplied in response to her distress. Following two falls in three weeks, the family members began to comprehend her increasing incapacity. Ella was lucid but simply seemed unable to muster the energy needed to function adequately. A housekeeper/companion was hired for 40 hours a week and family members began taking turns staying with her at night. Ella enjoyed this increased attention and became even more dependent to ensure it would remain. Within a few weeks, the family members began bickering about whose turn it was to stay as they became frustrated and angry about the increasing dependency of their mother. Ella was sensitive to how each member would respond to her demands and was therefore apparently not consistent in her behavior. Janet was irritated because Ella frequently called out at night but didn't do so when her sister, Laura, stayed overnight. Janet didn't recognize her irritation as associated with suppressed feelings that Laura had always been mother's favorite. Janet was 55 years old and beginning to be aware of her own aging and envious of Laura, 10 years younger. In addition, Laura was lighthearted and always could make Ella laugh while Janet was the one who always had to deal with the problems. Deep bitterness was seething in Janet.

It is apparent that some difficult decisions face this family. There are no right answers; there are none that will make everyone happy. Most significantly the social worker, nurse, or doctor who interviews/ counsels this family must appreciate the influence of a long and complex family history. In this respect, individual bias must be considered; reports from one individual cannot be taken at face value unless balanced against others.

In addition, elders who feel a threat to their independence will tend to overestimate their abilities. The following example illustrates this tendency.

> Art had been in a state mental institution most of his adult life and was transferred to a nursing home in 1970, near the community of his two elder sisters. Their interactions over the years had consisted of an exchange of cards and gifts for special occasions and holiday dinners together. This level of interaction continued in spite of his geographic relocation considerably nearer the family home and though he felt able to go home, Art and his sisters seemed mutually resigned to sustain the long-standing familiar patterns of infrequent but reliable contact within the relationship though Art was deeply disappointed.

Spouses typically exert great caregiving efforts to prevent institutionalization of a partner even to the detriment of their own health. When they are finally forced by ill health or depletion of energy to seek placement for the spouse, they may see it as a personal failure, even unethical. Often, when younger and in good health, each promised never to put the other "in a home." Promises made in the heat of passion or the confidence of youth and health unfortunately bind the psyche at other, less propitious, times. Also, when feeling personally threatened, the indisposed spouse is not above reminding the other of that promise.

When the family caregiver has reached the "end of the rope" or the "last straw" has caused total collapse, decisions are made in haste and in a crisis mode. Wolanin and Phillips (1981) speak of developing sets of contingency plans to avoid making hasty, inappropriate decisions. It is useful for professional caregivers to discuss this with family members and elders when they are not under pressure and can make wise decisions.

While there exists voluminous literature regarding the role of families in the care of elders in the community, it is much less clear what is expected or possible when the individual is in the hospital or a long-term care facility. Often, family members tend to criticize institutional care directly proportionate to the level of abandonment guilt they feel. While this belief may help professionals deal with the criticism of care heard from family members, it does nothing to assuage the indictments. At this time, given the awareness of the individuality of families and the overriding influence of family history, caregivers can only and with some temerity:

Get to know the family and their needs and fears.
Identify the power base within the family.
Determine the family member's hopes and expectations regarding the elder individual.
Provide opportunities for families to meet and discuss mutual problems.
Give feedback regarding the individual's appreciation of family attention.
Provide *private* time for family to visit.
Develop a list of useful behaviors to be given to all families when a member is admitted.
Enlist family assistance and input whenever feasible.

Services commonly provided by family to institutionalized elders include:

Grooming assistance.
Bringing things such as food, money, flowers, books, and clothing.
Straightening drawers and closets.
Taking resident on walks and outings.
Taking care of resident's laundry.
Making special occasions (such as birthdays) really special.
Assisting with feeding when necessary.

It is equally important to assist residents to identify ways in which they can add quality and meaning to visits from significant others. Some of the following issues could be the content of group discussions related to entertaining visitors in an institutional environment:

Giving specific positive feedback.
Avoiding guilty accusations.
Recording and sharing family history.
Cultivating listening skills.
Becoming more assertive.
Discussing difficult subjects: death, finances, illness.

Many families avoid talking about unpleasant events in an effort to protect the elder from worry. In reality, however, such avoidance pushes the elder to the periphery of the family and reduces him or her to a symbolic role. Below is an example that illustrates this process.

Grace had not been visited by her daughter for three weeks though the daughter had, prior to that, been consistent in visiting every week. Grace's granddaughter had heroically been protecting her from the news that Grace had been hospitalized and diagnosed as having breast cancer. Grace's lucidity had noticeably deteriorated over the last few weeks and the granddaughter felt that protecting Grace from the truth was kind. However, she never realized that her grandmother's deterioration was directly related to her anxiety and awareness of something amiss but her lack of knowledge of the actual problem.

Conversely, Eleanor was moderately demented and resided in the residential section of a nursing home. Her husband, who had been in the same facility but in the skilled nursing area, died. She attended the memorial service for him and expressed her grief at various times but it was hard for her to remember that he was gone. Occasionally she would return to the room he had occupied in the skilled nursing section of the facility and search for him. The nurses were patient with her and told her each time that he had died but they knew how much she missed him and it was alright for her to come to the unit to talk with them. She would then return to her area of the facility, seemingly content. She dealt with her grief and continued to function as she had before he died. She did not fully comprehend his death at all times but in her own way she managed to cope, even with her limited cognitive capacities.

Family members have a difficult time following the fine line of acceptable interaction in the institution. If they are heavily involved, they may be accused of interfering and if they are not visible or articulate in voicing their concerns they may be seen as disinterested and having abdicated their spousal or filial responsibility. According to Brody (1985), this places families in the classic "Catch-22" bind.

Amid the welter of opinions about the family's role in the care of the institutionalized elder, the opinion of the elder is notable by its absence. What does the aged person want from family at this time? What does the aged person think is realistic to expect from family members at this time? In what ways are the expectations of family members congruent with those of the elder? An example of assumptions being made without asking the elder is presented below.

Eloise needed to find a protective setting for her parents, both in their 90s. It took considerable time and investigation to find a setting that seemed suitable for the couple and provided sufficient monitoring for them to continue semi-independent living. Upon their arrival, Eloise was dismayed when her mother refused to share a room with her husband. She stoutly proclaimed she had lived with him for 60 years and she would now like a place of her own.

FAMILY AS CLIENT

Brody (1985) proposes the following issues as pertinent to the mental health of families with institutionalized elders:

- Mitigation of the negative effects of "placing" a family member.
- Identify, clarify, augment, and enhance positive role changes of family that occur in response to institutionalization of member.
- Clarify role perception and expectations family have of staff and resident.
- Assist family members to identify feasible involvement in facility that will give them satisfaction.
- Are there particular ethnic/cultural values that must be given special attention by staff or family?

The efforts of all health care professions will be needed to enhance the roles of families in relation to their elderly relatives who reside in nursing homes.

SURROGATE FAMILY CAREGIVERS

As mentioned earlier, 10% or more of institutionalized elders have no one designated as next-of-kin. Some or all of the various family services previously mentioned may be lacking in the lives of residents without families.

In some cases, residents are "geriatric orphans" who have outlived all family members and have no significant person left who has a shared life history. Caregivers really don't know, can barely even imagine, how this affects the sense of self that is continually reinforced and elaborated by the reflected appraisal of significant others. The nourishment of personal identity that occurs spontaneously and routinely is normally eroded in any institutional setting. However, it may be entirely lost to the geriatric orphan. It is as if, for the geriatric orphan, the radar "blip" has disappeared and contact with one's "ground" is lost.

Caregivers have effectively used focused group reminiscing to relieve some feelings of isolation and abandonment experienced by the geriatric orphan. To supply the missing affective sustenance and identity affirmation usually obtained from family, the group leader will need to consider certain guidelines:

Provide frequent verbal and nonverbal affective confirmation.
Guide discussion to commonly experienced life events.
Reinforce both individual and collective experience.
Enhance a sense of "belonging" by closed membership and group stability.
A criterion of group membership is no next-of-kin.

All of the principles of group reminiscence are applicable to these groups with particular attention to anything that will enhance the feeling of togetherness, shared experience, belonging, continuity, and caring that are usually the function of family. The more pragmatic functions that are noted in Chapter 4 may be thoughtfully examined to determine ways in which the group might also fulfill some of these functions. For instance, in personal care residents may assist each other with hair styling or selecting clothing for the day; if given assertiveness guidance and support, participation in decision making is also an effective way to use the group. For example, when Eleanor was told she could not save perishable food in her room, the group helped her propose a reasonable compromise and one group member accompanied her to talk to the administrator.

When others in the facility are attending family night, the "orphans" will attend a group with surrogate family.

CONCLUSION

This chapter has addressed family caregivers, their patterns of care, some aspects of home care, care of the Alzheimer's victim, and issues pertinent to institutionalization of a family member. For additional insight into the history and deficiencies in home care Mundinger's (1983) overview is recommended.

Epilogue: Future Trends

Future directions in providing for the mental health of the aged will be influenced by general social trends, reimbursement policies, education of mental health professionals, directions in mental health care of the total population, and models of care delivery.

Issues unique to the aged are based on demographics, however. Jones (1980, pp. 1–9) has noted the most significant demographic factor is the "passage of the pig through the python." This is the population bulge formed by "baby boomers," children born in the 1940s and 1950s that have formed social trends by the sheer pressure of their size and needs. They will reach retirement age and begin needing resources to support certain degrees of dependency between the years 2010 and 2040. Health and welfare resources in both economic and human terms must be enlisted in greater amounts than ever before to address their needs. As a result, shifts in spending priorities and reassessment of the way in which the health care dollar is distributed must come about. Some say rationing or coupons will be necessary; others believe preventive health care and the general level of health consciousness of this group will decrease the need for certain kinds of services.

As in the past, families will remain the chief support of elders. However, as young and mid-life adults have tended to have fewer children and will live longer, the burden of care they will place on their families may be more intense. Undoubtedly, there will be more education and support services directed toward reinforcing family responsibility. Caregivers expect tax deductions and expanded respite care resources will ease some of the stress. There is also evidence that churches and corporations are assuming more responsibility for the needs of families within their pale. Caregivers can expect them to become more directly involved and effective in this respect.

Young persons will need to begin early planning for old age and invest in some type of long-term care insurance. Given the fiscal disasters of Medicare, it is doubtful that long-term care insurance will be publicly financed but will most likely continue to be a private insurance venture. Caregivers will also see in the near future that those who lack family, personal, and economic resources will continue to be warehoused, abused, or left to wander homeless in the inner cities.

Preparation of professional caregivers devoted to working with the aged has increased enormously. In less than two decades, almost every university, college, and community college has included some type of education related to gerontology and the needs of the aged. Geropsychiatric specialties are still rather rare but caregivers should look for a great increase in this emphasis. Caregivers must remember the "baby boomers" have grown up in a "psychologized" environment and will seek and expect care of their mental health as well as physical health care.

Increasingly, mental health care will be provided through group participation and brief hospitalizations when necessary. Employee assistance programs will be designed to respond more effectively to the mental health of aging workers and will provide more support services to enhance preretirement years. Organic dementias that contribute so greatly to the long-term institutionalization of persons with mental aberrations may be more wisely treated and perhaps prevented. Much research has gone into attempts to discover the cause and cure of Alzheimer's disease and related disorders. Caregivers can reasonably expect marked progress in the near future.

Ethical decisions will command more attention as perceptive individuals continue to question the consistency and wisdom of health care decisions made on an individual, local, and national level. Mental health issues are particularly at the mercy of these decisions as they affect quality of life and capacity for seeking satisfaction. Many of the assaults on mental health are of an economic nature and are influenced by policies and restrictions over which one may have little control. Other emotional problems are the direct result of the way health care is presently decided and provided. Caregivers expect the upcoming generation of aged individuals to be much more vociferous about their needs than previous generations, as they have habitually made their voice heard in society.

Women's issues are becoming more of a focal point in planning services and mental health care as the nature of their experience and expectations has changed drastically in only a few decades. Women will no longer placidly accept diagnoses based on a male-dominated and defined nomenclature. There is also increasing awareness of the frequency with which a female spouse essentially sacrifices herself to the needs of her husband yet has no one to assist her when she can no longer manage. As a result, younger women are less likely to continue these patterns, particularly as many have been single parents and may have had a series of intimate relationships but none with whom they wish to devote the energies of their later years.

The needs of the future are slowly beginning to be met. The Omnibus Reconciliation Act of 1987 (OBRA-87) is a federal action that will significantly affect the type and quality of care provided to mentally ill patients in nursing homes. Clear directions are still needed to determine the full impact of this new legislation.

Finally, caregivers have already seen and can expect further evidence of the erosion of ageism. The more positive view of aging that is portrayed in the arts, humanities, and in much of our media has produced more general awareness of the uniqueness and diversity of the aged. The problems of the aged are also continually brought to our attention through media and personal exposure. It seems that as a society we are maturing. We are now able to see more clearly than ever before the complexity of the issues before us. We know that our own future in an aging society must be dealt with now.

References

Aasen, N. (1987). Interventions to facilitate personal control. *Journal of Gerontological Nursing, 13*(6), 21-27.

Addonzio, G. (1987). Neuroleptic malignant syndrome: A potentially fatal complication of neuroleptic use in elderly patients [Abstract]. *Proceedings of the 3rd Congress of the International Psychogeriatric Association, 3,* 5.

American Association of Retired Persons. (1986). Miles away and still caring: A guide for long-distance caregivers. Washington, DC: Author.

American Association of Retired Persons. (1987). Resources for caregivers. Washington, DC: Author.

American Psychiatric Association. (1987). *Diagnostic and statistical manual of mental disorders (3rd Ed-Revised).* Washington, DC: Author.

American Psychiatric Association. (1980). *Diagnostic and statistical manual of mental disorders (3rd Ed).* Washington, DC: Author.

Ancill, J. R. (1986). The grey area of geropsychiatry: Pseudodementia. *Gerontion,* 1(2), 16-19.

Annerstedt, L. (1987). Effects of an alternative mode of care for the demented elderly [Abstract]. *Proceedings of the 3rd Congress of the International Psychogeriatric Association, 3,* 61.

Bach, G., & Goldberg, H. (1974). *Creative aggression.* New York: Doubleday.

Baldwin, B. (1987). Innovations in mental health training programs for nursing home staff [Abstract]. *Proceedings of the 3rd Congress of the International Psychogeriatric Association, 3,* 87.

Bahr, S. R. T., & Gress, L. (1985). The 24 hour cycle: Rhythms of healthy sleep (developing nursing strategies). *Geriatric Nursing, 11*(4), 14-17.

247

Bayer, M., Bresloff, L., & Curley, D. (1986). The enhancement project: A program to improve the quality of resident's lives. *Geriatric Nursing*, 7(4), 192–195.
Beck, A. (1970). Cognitive therapy: Nature and relation to depression. *Behavior therapy*, 1, 184–200.
Beck, A., & Beck, R. (1972). Screening depressed patients in family practice: A rapid technique. *Post Graduate Medicine*, 52, 81–85.
Beck, A. T., Rusk, A. J., Shaw, B. F., & Emery, G. (1979). *Cognitive theory of depression*. New York: Guilford Press.
Beck, A., Ward, C., Mendelson, M., Mock, J., & Erbaugh (1961). An inventory for measuring depression. *Archives of General Psychiatry*, 4, 53–63.
Berezin, M. (1983). Psychotherapy in the elderly. In D. Breslau and M. Haug (Eds.), *Depression and aging: Causes, care, and consequences*. New York: Springer.
Berkman, L. & Syme, L. (1979). Social networks, host resistance, and mortality: A nine-year follow up study of Alameda County residents. *American Journal of Epidemiology*, 109, 186.
Berlinger, W., & Spector, R. (1984). Adverse drug reactions in the elderly. *Geriatrics*, 39, 45–58.
Bettis, S. (1979). Depression: The "common cold" of the elderly. *Generations 3*, 15, Spring.
Boettcher, E. (1983). Preventing violent behavior. *Perspectives in Psychiatric Care XXI*, 2, 54–58.
Boise Senior Center (1983). *Now my soul has elbow room: writings on healing*. Boise, ID: Boise Council on Aging.
Bolin, S. (1987). A comparative investigation of the effects of companion animals during conjugal bereavement [Abstract]. *Proceedings of the 3rd Congress of the International Psychogeriatric Association*, 3, 5.
Bond, C., & Miller, M. (1987, July/August). Reading: The ageless activity. *Geriatric Nursing*. 8(4), 192–193
Bootzin, R., & Shadish, W. (1986). Assessment and treatment in nursing homes: Implications for research. In M. Harper & B. Lebowitz (Eds.), *Mental health in nursing homes: Agenda for research*. Rockville, MD: US Department of Health and Human Services. DHHS Pub. No. (ADM) 86-1459.
Borden, W., Frankel, R., & Gierl, B. (1987). Stress and adaptation in chronic dementia: Predictors of well-being in family caregivers [Abstract]. *Proceedings of the 3rd Congress of the International Psychogeriatric Association*, 3, 12.
Borson, S. (1987). Secondary depression in the medically ill [Abstract]. *Proceedings of the 3rd Congress of the International Psychogeriatric Association*, 3, 133.
Boylin, W., Gordon, S., & Nehrke, M. (1976). Reminiscing and ego integrity in institutionalized elderly males. *Gerontologist*, 16(2), 118–124.
Brauer, W. (1987). A psychological caregiving approach to the cognitively impaired older adult, (Abstract). Chicago: *Proceedings of the 3rd Congress of the International Psychogeriatric Association*, 3, 19.
Brink, T. (1976). Geriatric counseling: A practical guide. *Family Therapy*, 3, 163.
Brink, T. (1984). Scale for assessing paranoia in the aged. *Clinical Gerontologist*, 3(2), 40.
Brink, T. et al. (1985, Fall). Geriatric depression scale reliability: Order, examiner and reminiscence effects. *Clinical Gerontologist*, 4, 57.
Brody, E. (1985). Parent care as a normative family stress. *Gerontologist*, 25(1), 19–29.
Bueber, M., & Hoffman, A. (1987). Perceived choice and resident satisfaction in a long-term care setting [Abstract]. *Proceedings of the 3rd Congress of the International Psychogeriatric Association*, 3, 52.

References   249

Burnside, I. (1973). *Psychosocial nursing care of the aged.* New York: McGraw-Hill.
Burnside, I. (1976). *Nursing and the aged.* New York: McGraw-Hill.
Burnside, I. (1984). *Working with the elderly: Group processes and techniques,* 2nd Ed. Belmont, CA: Wadsworth.
Butler, R. (1963). The life-review: An interpretation of reminiscence in the aged. *Psychiatry, 26,* 65–76.
Butler, R., & Lewis, M. (1982). *Aging and mental health,* 3rd Edition. St. Louis: C.V. Mosby. p. 315.
Byrd, R. (1938). *Alone.* New York: G. P. Putnam's.
Callahan, D. (1985). Feeding the dying elderly. *Generations, IX*(2), 15–17.
Casey, R., Masuda, M., & Holmes, T. (1967). Quantitative study of recall of life events. *Journal of Psychosomatic Research,* 11, 239–247.
Chenitz, C. (1979). Family support groups in nursing homes. Paper presented at the annual meeting of the *Western Gerontological Society,* March, Denver.
Clarfield, A. (1987). The reversibility of treatable dementia [Abstract]. *Proceedings of the 3rd Congress of the International Psychogeriatric Association,* 3, 54.
Cluff, P. (1975). The social corridor: An environmental and behavioral evaluation. *Gerontologist,* 15, 516.
Colby, K. (1977). Appraisal of four psychological theories of paranoid phenomena. *Journal of Abnormal Psychology,* 86, 54–59.
Connelly, B. (1987). Pet therapy for Alzheimer's disease [Abstract]. Chicago: *Proceedings of the 3rd Congress of the International Psychogeriatric Association.*
Cousins, N. (1979). *Anatomy of an illness.* New York: W. W. Norton.
Cowling, J. (1986, March). Health concerns of aging men. *Nursing Clinics of North America,* 21(1), 75–83.
Craven, S. (1988). Personal communication. San Francisco: Hillhaven Convalescent Care Facility.
Crook, T., Ferris, S., & McCarthy, M. (1979). The misplaced-objects task: A brief test for memory dysfunction in the aged. *Journal of the American Geriatric Society,* 27, 284–287.
Cuizon-Saiz, E. (1988). Personal communication. Anaheim, CA: Hillhaven Convalescent Hospital.
Dagon, E., & Van Sickle, A. (1987). Good grief: The development of time limited grief support groups in training gero-psychiatrists [Abstract]. *Proceedings of the 3rd Congress of the International Psychogeriatric Association,* 3, 130.
Dehlin, O., Agrell, B., Liden, A., Moser, G., & Olsen, I. (1987). Alprazolam: pharmacokinetics and clinical effect in the treatment of geriatric patients with neurotic depression [Abstract]. *Proceedings of the 3rd Congress of the International Psychogeriatric Association,* 3, 25.
Deitrich, C. (1986). *Assessment of the person with a behavioral problem.* San Francisco: University of California.
Dennis, H. (1978). Remotivation Therapy Groups. In I. Burnside (Ed.), *Working with the elderly: Group processes and techniques.* North Scituate, MA: Duxbury.
Donat, D. (1986). Altercations among institutionalized psychogeriatric patients. *Gerontologist,* 26(3), 227–228.
Dye, C. (1985). *Assessment and intervention in geropsychiatric nursing.* Orlando: Grune and Stratton.
Ebersole, P. (1976). The therapeutic value of reminiscing with the aged. *American Journal of Nursing,* 76, 601–602.
Ebersole, P. (1978a). A theoretical approach to the use of reminiscence. In

I. Burnside (Ed.), *Working with the elderly: Group processes and techniques.* No. Scituate, MA: Duxbury.

Ebersole, P. (1978b). Establishing reminiscing groups. In I. Burnside (Ed.), *Working with the elderly: Group processes and techniques.* North Scituate, MA: Duxbury.

Ebersole, P. (1986). Commitment to clinical excellence in nursing homes. In *Overcoming the bias of ageism in long term care.* New York: National League of Nursing.

Ebersole, P. (1988a). Nursing 209: Psychiatric Nursing Clinical Experience. Burlingame, CA: Mills-Peninsula Hospital.

Ebersole, P. (1988b). Personal experiences with students from San Francisco State University, Department of Nursing.

Ebersole, P. (1979). In Burnside, I., Ebersole, P., & Monea, H. *Caring and caretaking throughout the life span.* New York: McGraw-Hill.

Ebersole, P., & Hess, P. (1981). *Toward healthy aging: Human needs and nursing response.* St. Louis: C.V. Mosby.

Ebersole, P., & Hess, P. (1985). *Toward healthy aging: Human needs and nursing response* (2nd Ed.). St. Louis: C.V. Mosby.

Ebersole, P., & Hess, P. (1990, in press). *Toward healthy aging: Human needs and nursing response,* 3rd Ed. St. Louis: C.V. Mosby.

Ekerdt, D. (1986). The busy ethic: Moral continuity between work and retirement. *Gerontologist, 26*(3), 239–244.

Eliasberg, S. (1987). Addressing mental health needs in the long-term care setting: Challenges and achievements of a geropsychiatric clinical specialist in nursing [Abstract]. *Proceedings of the 3rd Congress of the International Psychogeriatric Association, 3,* 128.

Engel, G. L. (1980). The clinical application of the biopsychosocial model. *American Journal of Psychiatry, 137,* 535–544.

Evans, L. (1987). Sundowner syndrome in the institutionalized elderly. *Journal of American Geriatric Society, 35,* 101–108.

Falcone, A. (1984). Care based on need. *Geriatric Nursing, 5*(8), 376–380.

Falcone, A. (1983). Comprehensive functional assessment as an administrative tool. *Journal of the American Geriatrics Society, 31*(11), 642–650.

Farran, C. (1987). Maintaining a flexible group program [Abstract]. *Proceedings of the 3rd Congress of the International Psychogeriatric Association, 3,* 112.

Farran, C. (1987). Selected issues in managing a geriatric psychiatric inpatient unit [Abstract]. *Proceedings of the 3rd Congress of the International Psychogeriatric Association, 3,* 80.

Field, M. (1979). Urinary incontinence in the elderly: An overview. *Journal of Gerontological Nursing, 5,* 12.

Finlayson, R., Hurt, R., Davis, L., & Morse, R. (1987). Psychosocial and behavioral correlates of late life alcoholism [Abstract]. *Proceedings of the 3rd Congress of the International Psychogeriatric Association, 3,* 4–5.

Fink, M., Green, M., & Bender, M. (1952). The face-hand test as a diagnostic sign of organic mental syndrome. *Neurology, 2,* 46–59.

Folstein, M., Folstein, S., & McHugh, P. (1975). Mini-mental state: A practical method for grading the cognitive state of patients for the clinician. *Journal of Psychiatric Research, 12,* 189–198.

Francis, G., & Baly, A. (1986). Plush animals: Do they make a difference? *Geriatric Nursing, 7*(3), 140–142.

Funk & Wagnall (1983). *Funk & Wagnalls Standard Dictionary.* Revised Gazetteer Copyright. New York: Harper & Row.

Gaffney, J. (1986). Toward a less restrictive environment. *Geriatric Nursing*, 7(2), 94–95.

Gallagher, D. (1983). Procedural and clinical issues in the study of outpatient elder depressives: Recruitment, assessment, intervention, prediction. *Gerontologist*, 23, 297, special issue.

Gallo, J., Reichel, W., & Andersen, L. (1988). *Handbook of geriatric assessment*. Rockville, MD: Aspen.

Gamroth, L. (1983). Personal communication. Mt. Angel, Oregon: Benedictine Nursing Center.

Genevay, B. (1986). Sexuality and older people. *Generations*, X(4), 58–60.

Georgemiller, R., & Maloney, H. (1984). Group life review and denial of death. *Clinical Gerontologist*, 2, 37–49.

German, P. S., & Kramer, M. (1986). Nursing home study of the Eastern Baltimore epidemiological catchment area study. In M. Harper & B. Lebowitz (Eds.), *Mental illness in nursing homes: Agenda for research* (pp. 27–40) (DHHS Pub. No. (ADM) 86-1459). Rockville, MD: National Institute of Mental Health.

Gill, D. (1980). *Quest: The Life of Elizabeth Kubler-Ross*. New York: Ballantine Books.

Gillan, W. (1983). The effects of progressive relaxation on anxiety levels in the elderly. *Gerontologist*, 23, 93. Special Issue.

Gillies, D. (1986). Patients suffering from memory loss can be taught self-care. *Geriatric Nursing*, 7(5), 257–261.

Glynn, A. (1986). The therapy of music. *Journal of Gerontological Nursing*, 12(1), 14.

Gochros, H. (1972). The sexually oppressed. *Social Work* 16, 3–23.

Golander, H. (1987). Under the guise of passivity. *Journal of Gerontological Nursing*, 13(2), 26–30.

Goldfarb, A., & Turner, H. (1953). Psychotherapy of aged persons. II. Utilization and effectiveness of "brief" therapy. *American Journal of Psychiatry*, 109, 916.

Gordon, A. (1987). The importance of being earnest: Training clinicians to work with elderly dying people [Abstract]. *Proceedings of the 3rd Congress of the International Psychogeriatric Association*, 3, 134.

Gordon, M. (1985). *Manual of nursing diagnosis 1984-1985*. New York: McGraw-Hill.

Gordon, J., Siegal, A., & Palmer, I. (1987). Myths that solace - the subjective world of demented people in institutions [Abstract]. *Proceedings of the 3rd Congress of the International Psychogeriatric Association*, 3, 134.

Groves, ., & Kucharski, ., (1978). Personality types and reactions to illness.

Gurland, B. (1976). The comparative frequency of depression in various adult age groups. *Journal of Gerontology*, 31, 283.

Haag, A., & Stuhr, U. (1987). Interface of medicine and psychiatry in geriatrics [Abstract]. *Proceedings of the 3rd Congress of the International Psychogeriatric Association*, 3, 6.

Haley, D. (1987). Measurement of burnout in nurses' aides and licensed practical nurses employed in skilled nursing homes [Abstract]. *Proceedings of the 3rd Congress of the International Psychogeriatric Association*, 3, 124.

Hallal, J. (1985). Nursing diagnosis: An essential step to quality care. *Journal of Gerontological Nursing*, 11(9), 35–38.

Harel, Z., & Noelker, L. (1978, November). *The impact of social integration on the well-being and survival of institutionalized aged*. Paper presented at the 31st annual meeting of the Gerontological Society of America, Dallas, TX.

Haring, C., Miller, C., Barnas, C., & Fleischaker, W. (1987). Suicide in the elderly (Abstract). Chicago: *Proceedings of the 3rd Congress of the International Psychogeriatric Association*, 3, 17.

Harper, M. S. (1986). Introduction. In M. S. Harper & B. D. Lebowitz (Eds.), *Mental illness in nursing homes: Agenda for research* (pp. 1–6) (DHHS Pub. No. (ADM) 86-1459). Rockville, MD: National Institute of Mental Health.

Health Care Financing Administration (1982). *The Medicare and Medicaid data handbook, 1981.* Washington, DC: U.S. Government Printing Office.

Hellen, C. (1986). *Coping and caring: Living with Alzheimer's disease.* Washington, DC: American Association of Retired Persons.

Hess, P. (1985a). Age related differences and health assessment. In P. Ebersole and P. Hess, *Toward healthy aging: Human needs and nursing response,* 2nd Ed. St. Louis, C. V. Mosby.

Hess, P. (1985b). Life support needs. In P. Ebersole and P. Hess, *Toward healthy aging: Human needs and nursing response,* 2nd Ed. St. Louis, C. V. Mosby.

Hilliard, I. (1987). The new role of chaplains in homes for seniors [Abstract]. *Proceedings of the 3rd Congress of the International Psychogeriatric Association, 3,* 81.

Hollinger, J. (1986, March). Communicating with the elderly. *Journal of Gerontological Nursing.* 12(3), 8–14.

Hotchkiss, T. (1982). *Gerontological nurse practitioners: The new professionals* (film). Boise, ID: Tri-Media Communications.

Husaini, R., Linn, J., Neser, H., Whitten-Stoval, R., & Miller, R. (1987). Age and gender differences in sociomedical correlates of depression [Abstract]. *Proceedings of the 3rd Congress of the International Psychogeriatric Association, 3,* 47.

Hussian, R. (1986). Severe behavioral problems. In L. Teri and P. Lewinsohn (Eds.), *Geropsychological assessment and treatment.* New York: Springer.

Hussian, R., & Davis, R. (1983). *Analysis of wandering behavior in institutionalized geriatric patients.* Paper presented at the meeting of the Association for Behavioral Analysis. Milwaukee, WI.

Jacobson, E. (1974). *Progressive relaxation.* Chicago: University of Chicago Press, Midway Reprint.

Jarvik, L., & Russell, D. (1979). Anxiety, aging and the third emergency reaction. *Journal of Gerontology, 34,* 197.

Johnston, J. (1987). Fall prevention responses in the elderly [Abstract]. *Proceedings of the 3rd Congress of the International Psychogeriatric Association, 3,* 30.

Jones, L. (1980). *Great expectations: America, the baby boom generation.* New York: Ballantine.

Jones, L. (1981). *Great expectations: America and the baby boom generation.* New York: Ballantine Books. pps. 1–9.

Kahn, R., Goldfarb, A., Pollack, M., & Peck, A. (1960). Brief objective measures for the determination of mental status in the aged. *American Journal of Psychiatry, 117,* 326–328.

Kane, R. & Kane, R. (1981). *Assessing the elderly: A practical guide to measurement.* Baltimore: Heath.

Kane, R., Bell, R., & Riegler, S. (1986). Value preferences for nursing home outcomes. *Gerontologist, 26(3),* 303–308.

Kane, R., Garrard, J., Buchanan, J., Arnold, M., Kane, R., & McDermott, S. (1988). *The geriatric nurse practitioner as a nursing home employee: Conceptual and methodological issues in assessing quality of care and cost effectiveness.* Research Project Report to the Health Care Financing Administration, Robert Wood Johnson Foundation, and the W. K. Kellogg Foundation. Minneapolis: University of Minnesota School of Public Health.

Kane, R., Ouslander, J., & Abrass, I. (1989). *Essentials of clinical geriatrics,* 2nd. edition. New York: McGraw-Hill. pp. 201–205.

Kato, M. (1987). Suicide in the elderly in Japan (Abstract). Chicago: *Proceedings of the 3rd Congress of the International Psychogeriatric Association, 3,* 32.

Kiernan, P. J. & Isaacs, J. B. (1981). Use of drugs by the elderly. *Journal of the Society of Medicine 74,* 196–200.

King, H. (1987). A community psychogeriatric clinic: A model [Abstract]. *Proceedings of the 3rd Congress of the International Psychogeriatric Association, 3,* 7.

Knight, R., Reinhart, R., & Field, P. (1982). Senior outreach services: A treatment oriented outreach team in community health. *Gerontologist, 22,* 544.

Koenig, H. (1987). Religion and well-being in later life. [Abstract]. *Proceedings of the 3rd Congress of the International Psychogeriatric Association, 3,* 81.

Kolata, G. (1982, December 17). Food affects human behavior. *Science, 218,* 1209–1210.

Kral, V., & Emery, O. (1987). Long term follow-up of depressive pseudodementia in the aged [Abstract]. *Proceedings of the 3rd Congress of the International Psychogeriatric Association, 3,* 30.

Kretschmar, C., & Wurthmann, C. (1987). Outcome of depression in old age [Abstract]. *Proceedings of the 3rd Congress of the International Psychogeriatric Association, 3,* 31.

Krieger, D. (1975). Therapeutic touch: The imprimatur of nursing. *American Journal of Nursing, 75,* 784.

Lardaro, T. (1987). Reactions of therapists to the death of elderly patients in psychotherapy [Abstract]. *Proceedings of the 3rd Congress of the International Psychogeriatric Association, 3,* 29–30.

Larocca, F. (1987). Eating disorders in the elderly: transgenerational psychiatry [Abstract]. *Proceedings of the 3rd Congress of the International Psychogeriatric Association, 3,* 5–6.

Lawton, M., & Storandt, M. (1984). Assessment of older people. In P. McReynolds & G. Chelune (Eds.), *Advances in psychological assessment* (Vol. 6). San Francisco: Jossey-Bass.

Lehr, U. (1987). Elderly daughters caring for their old parents [Abstract]. *Proceedings of the 3rd Congress of the International Psychogeriatric Association, 3,* 5.

Levine, S. (1983). Dying at home. *Medical Self-Care, 2,* 14.

Levitan, S. J., & Kornfeld, D. S. (1981). Clinical and cost benefits of liaison psychiatry. *American Journal of Psychiatry, 138,* 790–793.

Libow, L. (1977). Pseudo-senility: Acute and reversible organic brain syndrome. In C. Eisdorfer and R. Friedel (Eds.), *Cognitive and emotional disturbance in the elderly: Clinical issues.* Chicago: Year Book Medical Pubs.

Lightfoot, O., & To, A. (1989). Long term followup of behavioral disorders in geriatric patients. New Orleans: Presentation at the National Council on Aging Conference.

Liptzin, B. (1986). Major mental disorders/problems in nursing homes: Implications for research and public policy. In M. Harper & B. Lebowitz (Eds.), *Mental illness in nursing homes: Agenda for research* (pp. 41–56) (DHHS Pub. No. (ADM) 86–1459). Rockville, MD: National Institute of Mental Health.

Loebel, J. (1987). Requests for psychiatric consultation in long term care facilities [Abstract]. *Proceedings of the 3rd Congress of the International Psychogeriatric Association, 3,* 32.

Long, R. (1962). Remotivation—Fact or fantasy. *Mental Hospital Service, 151,* 1–8.

Lowenthal, M. & Haven, C. (1968). Interaction and adaptation: Intimacy as a critical variable. *American Sociologic Review, 33,* 20.

Lund, C., & Shafer, R. (1985). Is your patient about to fall? *Journal of Gerontological Nursing, 11*(4), 37–41.

Luthe, W. (1963). Autogenic training: Method, research and application. *American Journal of Psychotherapy, 1963, 17,* 174–195.

Mace, N. (1983). Speech at Geriatric Regional Education Center (GREC). Boise, ID: Veterans Admin. Medical Center.

Mace, N., & Rabins, P. (1984). Day care and dementia. *Generations, 9*(2), 41–45.

Mace, N. L., & Rabins, P. V. (1981). *The 36-hour day.* Baltimore, MD: The Johns Hopkins Press.

Maddox, G., Robins, L., & Rosenberg, N. (1986). *Nature and extent of alcohol problems among the elderly.* New York: Springer.

Manderino, M., & Bzdek, V. (1986). Mobilizing depressed clients. *Journal of Psychosocial Nursing, 24*(5), 23–28.

Marshall, J. (1978). Changes in aged white male suicide: 1948–1972. *Journal of Gerontology, 33,* 763.

Martens, K. (1986). Let's diagnose strength, not just problems. *American Journal of Nursing, 86*(2), 192–193.

Maslow, A. (1970). *Motivation and personality.* (2nd Ed). New York: Harper & Row.

Masuda, M., & Holmes, T. H. (1967). Magnitude estimations of social readjustments. *Journal of Psychosomatic Research, II,* 219–225.

Matthiesen, V. (1987). Adult daughters' relationship with their institutionalized mothers [Abstract]. *Proceedings of the 3rd Congress of the International Psychogeriatric Association, 3,* 23.

McCracken, A. (1987). Emotional impact of possession loss. *Journal of Gerontological Nursing, 13*(2), 14–18.

McNulty, E., & Dann, M. (1984). *The dilemma of caring.* Springfield, IL: Charles C. Thomas.

Mead, M. (1972). *Blackberry winter: My earlier years.* New York: Morrow.

Miller, M. (1978). Note: Toward a profile of the older white male suicide. *Gerontologist, 18,* 80–84.

Miller, S. (1986). Relationships in long-term care facilities. *Generations, X*(4), 65–67.

Milton, I., & MacPhail, J. (1985). Dolls and toy animals for hospitalized elders—infantalizing or comforting? *Geriatric Nursing, 6*(4), 204–206.

Mintzer, J., D'Elia, L., Mintz, J., Small, G., & Jarvik, L. (1987). Are symptoms of anxiety and depression related in geriatric patients? [Abstract]. *Proceedings of the 3rd Congress of the International Psychogeriatric Association, 3,* 28.

Monea, H. (1978). *Peer counseling: Perspectives in learning with the older adult.* San Francisco: Commission on Aging.

Morganette, B. (1987, July/August). Nature hikes for nursing home residents. *Geriatric Nursing, 8*(4), 178–179.

Morse, J., Tylko, S., & Dixon, H. (1987). Characteristics of the fall prone patient. *Gerontologist, 27*(4), 516–522.

Mundinger, M. (1983). *Home care controversy: Too little, too late, too costly.* Rockville, MD: Aspen.

Murray, R. B. (1984). Model for psychiatric and mental health nursing: Negative self-concept. In Carlson, Kraft, McGuire (Eds.), *Nursing diagnosis: Client models for utilization.* New York: W. B. Saunders, Co.

National Center for Health Statistics (1983). *An overview of the 1980 national master facility inventory survey of nursing and related homes.* (Advance Data #91. DHHS Pub. No. (PHS) 83-1250). Hyattsville, MD: Public Health Service.

Naughton, B. (1987). Medical disease presentation as psychiatric illness [Abstract]. *Proceedings of the 3rd Congress of the International Psychogeriatric Association, 3,* 127.

Nesbit, D. (1987). Attitudinal barriers to delivery of mental health services to the elderly [Abstract]. *Proceedings of the 3rd Congress of the International Psychogeriatric Association, 3*, 16.

Neugarten, B. (1968). Adult personality: Toward a psychology of the life cycle. In B. Neugarten (Ed.), *Middle age and aging*. Chicago: University of Chicago Press.

Nick, S. (1987). Quality of life nursing care: outcomes for nursing home residents [Abstract]. *Proceedings of the 3rd Congress of the International Psychogeriatric Association, 3*, 80.

Norberg, A., Athlin, E., & Asplund, K. (1987). Feeding problems in severely demented patients (Abstract). Chicago: *Proceedings of the 3rd Congress of the International Psychogeriatric Association, 3*, 64.

Norris, C. (1986). Restlessness: A disturbance in rhythmicity. *Geriatric Nursing 7*, 6, 20.

O'Connor, C. (1987). Psychosocial aspects of care with elderly veterans by a gerontological clinical specialist in a United States veterans administration hospital [Abstract]. *Proceedings of the 3rd Congress of the International Psychogeriatric Association, 3*, 111.

O'Connor, C. (1985). *Aggression as communication*. Paper presented at Geropsychiatric Conference, Levindale Hebrew Home. Baltimore, MD.

Older American Reports (1983). 7:5, June 24. Washington D.C. Capital Publishers.

Oppeneer, J., & Vervoren, T. (1983). *Gerontological pharmacology: A resource for health practitioners*. St Louis: C. V. Mosby.

Osis, M. (1986). Insomnia in the elderly: Sleeping pills or warm milk? *Gerontion 1*(3), 8–11.

Ostrovski, M. (1980). *Alleviation of depression through group reminiscing*. Unpublished master's thesis. Lone Mountain College, San Francisco, CA.

Ouslander, J. G. (1981). Urinary incontinence in the elderly. *Western Journal of Medicine, 135*, 482–491.

Parsons, C. (1986). Group reminiscence therapy and levels of depression in the elderly. *Nurse Practitioner, 11*(3), 68–76.

Patterson, R. L., & Jackson, G. M. (1980). Behavior modification in the elderly. In M. Hersen, R. Eisler, & P. Miller (Eds.), *Progress in behavior modification, 9*. New York: Academic Press.

Pomerantz, R., & Meyer, R. (1987). Hypothyroidism in the elderly: A frequently unsuspected clinical entity [Abstract]. *Proceedings of the 3rd Congress of the International Psychogeriatric Association, 3*, 39.

Power, S. (1986). A nutritional challenge: The elderly patient with dysphagia. *Gerontion, 1*(2), 12–13.

Psychiatric Nursing Phenomena Task Force. (1986). *Psychiatric Nursing Diagnoses*. Kansas City, MO: American Nurses' Association.

Rabins, P. (1987). Depression in old and young: is it different? (Abstract). Chicago: *Proceedings of the 3rd Congress of the International Psychogeriatric Assocation, 3*, 8.

Rader, J., Doan, J., & Schwab, M. (1985). How to decrease wandering, a form of agenda behavior. *Geriatric Nursing, 6*, 196–199.

Rahe, R. (1972). Subject's recent life changes and their near-future illness reports. *Annals of Clinical Research, 4*, 250–265.

Reifler, B. V. (1986). Alzheimer's disease in nursing homes: Current practice and implications for research. In M. Harper & B. Lebowitz (Eds.), *Mental health in nursing homes: Agenda for research* (DHHS Pub. No. (ADM) 86-1459). Rockville, MD: National Institute of Mental Health.

Reifler, B., Larson, E., Cox, G., & Featherstone, H. (1981). Treatment results at a multi-specialty clinic for the impaired elderly and their families. *Journal of the American Geriatrics Society, 29,* 579–582.

Richards, M. (1986). Relationship Bridges in nursing homes: Family support groups. *Generations,* X(4), 68–70.

Richards, W. S., & Thorpe, G. L. (1978). Behavioral approaches to the problems of later life. In M. Storandt, I. Siegler, & M. Elias (Eds.), *The clinical psychology of aging.* New York: Plenum Press.

Rodin, J., & Langer, E. (1977). Long term effects of a control-relevant intervention with the institutionalized aged. *Journal of Personality and Social Psychology, 35,* 897–902.

Rovner, B. (1987). Prevalence of mental disorders in nursing homes: health service needs and allocation of resources [Abstract]. *Proceedings of the 3rd Congress of the International Psychogeriatric Association, 3,* 93.

Roy, B., Obaid, M., and Rudick, S. (1987). Pattern of psychiatric illness in elderly and the role of a mobile geriatric treatment team - management outcome and cost effectiveness [Abstract]. *Proceedings of the 3rd Congress of the International Psychogeriatric Association, 3,* 9.

Rubin, E., Devverts, W., & Burke, W. (1987). Psychotic symptoms in the course of senile dementia of the Alzheimer's type (Abstract). Chicago: *Proceedings of the 3rd Congress of the International Psychogeriatric Association, 3,* 160.

Rugh, M. (1987). Art therapy with institutionalized older adults [Abstract]. *Proceedings of the 3rd Congress of the International Psychogeriatric Association, 3,* 3.

Sakauye, K. (1986). Interface of emotional and behavioral conditions with physical disorders in nursing homes. In M. Harper & B. Lebowitz (Eds.), *Mental health in nursing homes: Agenda for research.* (DHHS Pub. No. (ADM) 86-1459). Rockville, MD: National Institute of Mental Health.

Sakauye, K., & McDonald, M. (1987). The impact of "caring touch" on quality of life in a nursing home (Abstract). Chicago: *Proceedings of the 3rd Congress of the International Psychogeriatric Association, 3,* 131.

Sands, D. (1983). Agitation and paranoid accusation: The role of precipitating incidents. *Clinical Gerontologist, 1,* 74–75.

Satir, V. (1972). *Peoplemaking.* Palo Alto, CA: Science and Behavior Books, Inc. pps 59–80.

Schafer, S. (1985). Modifying the environment. *Geriatric Nursing,* 6(3), 157–159.

Schaffer, C., & Donlon, P. (1983). Medical causes of psychiatric symptoms in the elderly. *Clinical Gerontologist,* 1(4), 3–17.

Schuman, J. (1987). Palliative care in a Catholic institution [Abstract]. *Proceedings of the 3rd Congress of the International Psychogeriatric Association, 3,* 82.

Schwartz, G. (1987). The role of family members in geriatric psychopharmacology [Abstract]. *Proceedings of the 3rd Congress of the International Psychogeriatric Association, 3,* 61.

Shomaker, D. (1987). Problematic behavior and the Alzheimer patient: Retrospection as a method of understanding and counseling. *Gerontologist,* 27(3), 370–373.

Sine, R. (1986, February). A lateralized stroke rehabilitation program for elderly patients. *3rd Annual Geriatrics Symposium.* San Francisco: Sponsored by St. Mary's Hospital and the American Heart Association. Reprinted from "Basic Rehabilitation Techniques" Boulder, Co: Aspen Publications.

Slimmer, L., Lopez, M., LeSage, J., & Ellor, J. (1987). Perceptions of learned helplessness. *Journal of Gerontological Nursing,* 13(5), 33–37.

Sloan, R. (1978). Psychiatric problems of the aged. Paper presented at the Comparative Psychiatric Therapies Conference, University of Southern California, Los Angeles.

Snyder, L., Rupprecht, P., & Pyrek, J. (1978). Wandering. *Gerontologist, 18*, 272–280.

Spencer, R., Nichols, L., Lipkin, G., Waterhouse, H., West, F., & Bankert, E. (1986). Drug therapy in gerontological nursing. In *Clinical Pharmacology and Nursing Management*, 2nd Ed. Philadelphia: J. B. Lippincott.

Spiegel, R. (1987). Sleep disorders in the elderly [Abstract]. *Proceedings of the 3rd Congress of the International Psychogeriatric Association, 3*, 90.

Stern, R. (1985). Staff development and communication with the aged. Workshop sponsored by Vista College and Hillhaven Corporation. Oakland, CA.

St. George, J., & DiCicco-Bloom, B. (1985). Using dramatization to train caregivers of the elderly. *Nursing Outlook, 33*(6), 302–304.

Stokes, S., & Gordon, S. (1988). Development of an instrument to measure stress in the older adult. *Nursing Research, 37*(1), 16–19.

Stotts, R. C., & Pickett, J. (1987). The camera as a nursing tool. *Geriatric Nursing, 8*, 130–132.

Suinn, R., & Richardson, F. (1971). Anxiety management training: A non-specific behavior therapy program for anxiety control. *Behavior Therapy, 2*, 498–510.

Sulkava, R., Haltia, M., Paetau, A., Wikstrom, J., & Palo, J. (1983). Accuracy of clinical diagnosis in primary degenerative dementia: Correlation with neuropathological findings. *Journal of Neurology, Neurosurgery, and Psychiatry, 46*, 9–13.

Talbot, M. (1987). Reactive depression in nursing home patients (Abstract). Chicago: *Proceedings of the 3rd Congress of the International Psychogeriatric Association, 3*, 106.

Taube, R., & Barrett, J. (1986). *Mental Health in the United States, 1985*. National Institute of Mental Health, United States Department of Health and Human Services. Washington, D.C.: U.S. Government Printing Office.

Taulbee, L., & Folsom, J. (1966). Reality orientation for geriatric patients. *Hospital and Community Psychiatry, 17*, 133–138.

Teri, L., & Lewinsohn, P. (1986). *Geropsychological assessment and treatment*. New York: Springer Publishing Co.

Todd, B. (1986). Drugs and the elderly: When the risks outweigh the benefits. *Geriatric Nursing, 7*(4), 212, 222.

Troyer, D. (1984). A "share your heart" program: benefits to patients and staff. *Journal of the American Health Care Association, 10*, 22–26.

Vanthooft, F. (1987). Phenomenology of dementia behavior (Abstract). Chicago: *Proceedings of the 3rd Congress of the International Psychogeriatric Association, 3*, 19.

Verstraten, P. (1987). The GIP: fourteen subscales for observing psychogeriatric inpatients [Abstract]. *Proceedings of the 3rd Congress of the International Psychogeriatric Association, 3*, 33.

Wasson, W., & Grunes, J. (1987). The dynamisms of depressive experience among women in late life [Abstract]. *Proceedings of the 3rd Congress of the International Psychogeriatric Association, 3*, 116.

Weber, G., & McCall, G. (1987). *The nursing assistant's casebook of elder care*. Dover, MS: Auburn House.

Weinstein, (1986, February). Aquatic activity benefits aging. *Journal of Gerontological Nursing, 12*(2), 6–11.

Weldon, S., & Yesavage, J. S. (1982). Behavioral improvement with relaxation training in senile dementia. *Clinical Gerontologist, 1*, 45–50.

Wells, T. (1982). What does commitment to gerontological nursing really mean? *Journal of Gerontological Nursing, 8*, 434–437.

Wells, T. (1982). *Aging and health promotion*. Rockville, MD: Aspen.

Wichita, C. (1977). The effect of reminiscing therapy on apathetic elderly. Unpublished master's thesis, College of Nursing, University of Arizona, Tucson, AZ.

Williams, H. (1986). Humor and healing: Therapeutic effects in geriatrics. *Gerontion,* 1(3), 14–17.

Wolanin, M. (1982). Personal communication. Tucson, AZ.

Wolanin, M. (1985). Personal communication. Tucson, AZ.

Wolanin, M., & Phillips, L. (1981). *Confusion: Prevention and Care.* St. Louis: C. V. Mosby.

Wolpe, J. (1969). *The practice of behavior therapy.* New York: Pergamon Press.

Wyler, A., Masuda, M., & Holmes, T. (1968). Seriousness of illness rating scale. *Journal of Psychosomatic Research,* 11, 363–374.

Yalom, I. (1970). *The theory and practice of group psychotherapy.* New York: Basic Books.

Yanchick, V. (1985). Drug therapy. In C. Dye (Ed.), *Assessment and intervention in Geropsychiatric Nursing.* Orlando: Grune and Stratton.

Yost, E. B., Beutler, L. E., Corbishley, M. A., & Allender, J. R. (1986). *Group cognitive therapy: A treatment approach for depressed older adults.* New York: Pergamon Press.

Zachow, K. (1984). Helen, can you hear me? *Journal of Gerontological Nursing,* 10, 18–22.

APPENDICES

APPENDIX A

Useful DSM-III-R Related to Nursing Diagnoses for Psychogeriatric Care

The following is a list of DSM III-R Classification categories most likely relevant to making a nursing diagnosis for aged clients with mental health problems:

Organic mental syndromes and disorders
    Nonsubstance induced
        Delirium
        Dementia
        Delusional syndrome
        Hallucinosis
        Affective syndrome
            Depressed
            Manic/agitated
        Anxiety/catastrophic reactions
        Personality syndrome
            Explosive

Primary degenerative dementia, senile onset
  (Alzheimer's disease and related disorders)
  Includes any of the above 2nd order manifestations
Multiinfarct dementia
  Strokes, Transient Ischemic attacks
  (CVAs and TIAs)
Organic mental disorders
  Substance induced
  Alcohol
    Dependence
    Withdrawal delirium
    Amnestic disorder
      (often accompanied by confabulation)
    Dementia
      (following long-term alcohol abuse)
    Barbiturates, sedatives, or hypnotics
    Dependence
    Withdrawal delirium
    Amnestic disorder
Sleep and arousal disorders
  Disorders of initiating or maintaining sleep
    Sleep-induced respiratory impairment
      Nonobstructive sleep apnea
      Nonapneic hypoventilation
        (both of the above may be medication induced)
      Chronic obstructive pulmonary disease (COPD)
    Insomnia or excessive daytime somnolence secondary to other
      physical disorders
    Subjective sleep disturbance without objective findings
  Disorders of the sleep–wake schedule
    Disorganized sleep–wake pattern
      (often in conjunction with delirium or advanced dementia)
Schizophrenic Disorders
  Schizophrenia
    Undifferentiated
      Late onset (usually mid-life crisis reaction)
Delusional S (Paranoid) disorders
  Somatic
  Persecutory
Mood (Affective) Disorders
  Depressive disorders
    Major depression
      Single episode or recurrent
    Dysthymia (anhedonia)

Anxiety Disorders
 Panic
  Without phobic avoidance
 Obsessive compulsive disorder
 Generalized anxiety disorder
Somatoform Disorders
 Somatization disorder
 Hypochondriasis (most often secondary to depression)
Gender and Sexual Disorders
 Sexual dysfunctions
  Sexual desire disorders
   Hypoactive sexual desire
  Sexual arousal disorders
   Male sexual arousal disorders
  Orgasm disorders
   Inhibited female orgasm
   Delayed or absent male orgasm (not listed)
  Sexual pain disorders
   Functional dyspareunia
   Functional vaginismus
    (both of the above related to infrequent intercourse, friable
     tissue, and hormone deficiencies)
Adjustment Disorder
  with depressed mood
  with anxious mood
  with withdrawal
  with physical complaints
Personality Disorders
 Paranoid
 Dependent
 Obsessive compulsive
 Passive aggressive
Conditions not attributable to a mental disorder
 Uncomplicated bereavement
 Phase of life problem or life circumstance
 Marital problem
 Parent–child problem
 Other specified family circumstances
 Other interpersonal problems

APPENDIX B

Sample Nursing Diagnosis Development for a Case of Depression

The following uses depression to examplify geropsychiatric nursing diagnosis development:

DSM-III-R: Affective Disorder: Major Depressive Episode: Single or Recurrent (Chronic is not listed but is often a reality): May be related to Adjustment Disorder or Conditions Not Attributable to a Mental Disorder

RESPONSE CLASS: I. INDIVIDUAL
   Response System: A. Biologic
   Nursing diagnoses: Alteration in bowel *elimination* related to:
      inactivity
      decreased peristalsis
      inadequate diet
      dehydration
      diminished tonus of involuntary muscles

Nursing diagnoses: Alteration in *nutrition* related to:
anorexia (most usual in profound depression)
excessive intake (usually related to boredom, attempts to fill the
    emptiness, reduced metabolic rate, and consumption of high
    caloric foods requiring little effort in preparation)
Nursing diagnoses: Alteration in *fluid volume* related to:
inattention to body cues
insufficient fluid intake
diminished respiration/perspiration
Nursing diagnoses: Potential for *infection* related to
self-neglect
nutritional deficits
endocrine response to stressors
Nursing diagnoses: Potential for *injury* related to:
impaired attention span
inattentive behaviors
confusion
disinterest
Response System: B. Behavioral
Nursing diagnoses: *Sexual* dysfunction related to:
decreased libido
bordeom/disinterest
decreased hormonal secretions
unavailability of partner
self-disgust
guilt
Nursing diagnoses: *Self-care* deficit related to:
decreased sense of worth
fatigue
indecisiveness
self-punishment
inattention to body
Nursing diagnoses: *Sleep pattern* disturbance related to:
early morning waking
overmedication
inactivity during waking hours
rumination about disappointments/failures
Nursing diagnoses: Potential for *violence* to self related to:
hopelessness/helplessness
physical deterioration
functional incapacity
decreased self-regard

debilitating disease
lingering fatal illness
Nursing diagnoses: Diversional *activity* deficit related to:
excessive dependence
psychomotor retardation
lethargy/fatigue
disinterest/boredom
withdrawal/isolation
inactivity
regression
Nursing diagnoses: Impaired *motor behavior* related to:
response lag
arousal deficit
muscle flaccidity
Nursing diagnoses: Impaired verbal *communication* related to:
inattention
thought slowing
poverty of thought
retreat from stimulation
interest deficit
Nursing diagnoses: Ineffective individual *coping* related to:
deterioration of usual coping mechanisms
physiological manifestations of persistent stress
fatigue
disinclination to meet basic needs
inability to make decisions
hypochondriasis
low self-esteem
Response System: C. Emotional
Nursing diagnoses: Impaired *range of expression* related to:
flattening of affect
apathy
feelings of worthlessness
absence of spontaneity
chronic grief
lability of affect
mood disturbance
Nursing diagnoses: Impaired *focus of expression* related to:
self-reproach
worthhlessness
despair
self-absorption

Nursing diagnoses: Impaired congruency of thoughts, behavior, and
emotions related to:
somatic preoccupation
hypochondriasis
Response System: D. Perceptual/Cognitive
Nursing diagnoses: Alterations in thought processes related to:
generalized *intellectual* slowing
withdrawal from intellectual stimulation
forgetfulness
memory impairment
    short term due to lack of attention
    long term recall negative distortions
    time disorientation
    time distortion
    confusion
judgment clouded by
    indecisiveness
    erosion of initiative
    avoidance of all risk
    negativism
    social isolation
thought processes
    impaired concentration
    impaired problem solving
    inattention
    poverty of ideas
    learning abilities slowed
thought content
    misinterpretations
    obsessions
    delusions of persecution (rare, primarily involutional)
    somatic delusions and hallucinations (primarily involutional)
    generalized pessimism
    ruminative
perceptions
    exaggeration of normal sensory changes of aging
        diminished hearing
        diminished vision
        loss of taste
        decreased kinesthetic awareness
        diminished interest in sensual experience
    sensory deprivation due to isolation

attention
    impaired concentration
    disinterest
    diminished attention span
orientation
    confusion
    disorientation, particularly to time

Response System: E. Value/Belief
Nursing diagnoses: Disturbance in *self-concept* related to:
    despair over meaninglessness
    alienation from self and beliefs
    alienation from others
    disappointment with life as lived
    apparent lack of justice
    spiritual issues
        demoralization
        guilt
        erosion of personal myths of
        invulnerability
        immortality
RESPONSE CLASS II. INTERPERSONAL/FAMILY
Response System: A. Identity/Interactional Processes
Nursing diagnoses: Impaired social *interactions* related to:
    disruption of *role structuring* through
        enforced disengagement
        selective disengagement
        role loss in response to
            death of significant other
            retirement
            relocation
            debilitating illness
        role reversal/disruption
        withdrawal
        dependence
    Affiliation
        exclusion through unpleasant/unacceptable behaviors such as:
            complaining
            ruminating
            demanding
            withholding
Nursing diagnoses: *Social isolation* related to:
    (internally or externally imposed?)

lack of energy to initiate activities
disinterest in events and activities
perceived stigmatization of self
lack of economic or transportational resources
insufficient attention to social network
alienating behaviors
Nursing diagnoses: Powerlessness related to:
perception of self and locus of control
disease processes not subject to individual control
knowledge deficits
institutional structures and expectations
inadequacy of resources
not being consulted regarding action/decisions
communication disorders
progressive debilitation
loss of function/abilities
ageism
unrealistic negative beliefs about capacities
Response System: B. Change/Stress Management
Nursing diagnoses: Ineffective family coping related to:
unproductive *conflict resolution*
exhaustion of caretakers
deference of own needs to depressed person
absence of satisfaction and relationship support
anger over excessive dependency of depressed person
respite resource deficits
reactivation of historic family problems
reliance on abuse/neglect/violence to manage frustration and despair
Nursing diagnoses: *Impaired grief* related to:
affiliative deficits
overwhelming losses
guilt
anger over abandonment
mythologizing the dead person
prolonged denial
Nursing diagnoses: *Grief reaction* related to:
recency of losses
process of resolution
individual modes of resolution
anticipation of loss
terminal illness
chronic pain
life-style change

Response System: C. Information Processing
Nursing diagnoses: Impaired home maintenance management related to:
inability to make decisions or concentrate
erosion of initiative
lack of energy/debilitation
distortion of *perceptions*
impairment of collective problem solving
preoccupation with individual rather than collective needs
inattention to surroundings
substance abuse
insufficient resources
inadequacy or exhaustion of support system
disturbed *communications*
RESPONSE CLASS: III. COMMUNITY/ENVIRONMENT/
AGGREGATE
Response System: A. Neighborhood/Community
Nursing diagnoses: Ineffective *family coping* related to:
inadequate resources for care
unconcerned/unavailable secondary supports
marginal institutions
unsafe neighborhood
knowledge deficits among health care providers
Response System: B. Environmental Stressors
Nursing diagnoses: Perceived powerlessness (individual/family/
group) related to:
national economic priorities
ageism
distribution priorities of limited health resources
stereotypic expectations culturally engendered
media portrayal of old age
euthanasia/dignified death
professional abuses of knowledge/authority

APPENDIX C

Gerontologic Pharmacologic Principles

Think of the following *Special Considerations*
Is there a low level of suspicion regarding negative effects of drugs?
Are there multiple prescribers?
Is there lack of inquiry into self-medication patterns?
Are there atypical symptoms: higher pain threshold, more referred pain?
Is there an ascription of symptoms to "old age"?
Is there insufficient attention to hearing, vision, understanding of information?
Was there insufficient time for adequate assessment?
Is there a narrow margin of homeostatic resilience?
Are there paradoxical reactions?

PHYSIOLOGIC CHANGES

Average changes in body mass increase accumulation of fat soluble drugs
    fluid decreases from 55 to 45% of body weight

hepatic function: most have normal metabolic function but certain drugs are significantly decreased; longer half-life results.
renal function: decreased renal blood flow, number of nephrons, glomerular filtration; results in drugs eliminated unchanged, remain in body longer, longer half-life in kidney
Reduced number or change in structure of drug receptors.
affect:
Absorption
Distribution
Metabolism
Elimination
Volume of distribution reduced; concentration higher
Produces greater competition for drug binding sites
Induces unpredicted drug interactions, e.g., congestive heart failure: normal adult dose may be toxic

PRINCIPLES OF GERIATRIC DRUG THERAPY

Is the drug necessary? Alternate therapies possible?
What is the therapeutic end point desired? Cure, relief, prolongation of life?
Is the drug correct? Misdiagnosis?
Is the dosage correct? More follow-up and titration needed:
Can't generalize dosage proportions, many dosages lower, some higher, such as antibiotics and diuretics.
Is the dosage form correct? Suppositories, liquids?
Compliance is often relative to form of drug.
What adverse side effects may occur?
Patient should be given information and education regarding orthostatic hypotension and other adverse reactions.
What drug interactions may occur? Drugs and foods to avoid.
Is the drug correctly labeled and packaged?
Can it be opened?
Is it in appropriate language?
Print large and legible?
Name, strength, quantity, dosage, name of client, name of prescriber clearly written?
Are major side effects listed?
Are activities, foods, and drugs to avoid listed?
Who is responsible for drug administration?
Are they capable?
Are they reliable?

Is the older person compliant? Noncompliance estimated from 20 to 80%. Need verbal and written instruction and return demonstration.

Can any medications be discontinued? When a drug is added, all other prescription and OTCs should be evaluated for discontinuation.

Adapted from: Pagliaro, L., & Pagliaro, A.(1983). *Pharmacologic aspects of aging*. St. Louis: C. V. Mosby.

APPENDIX D

Assessment Bibliography

GENERAL

Gallo, J., Reichel, W., & Anderson, L. (1988). Handbook of geriatric assessment. Rockville, MD: Aspen.

Kane, R., & Kane R. (1981). Assessing the elderly: A practical guide to measurement. Lexington, Massachusetts: Lexington Books.

ACTIVITIES OF DAILY LIVING

1. ADL's
Katz, S., Ford, A. B., Moskowitz, R. W., Jackson, B. A., & Jaffee, M. W. (1963). Studies of illness in the aged. Journal of the American Medical Association, 94ff
2. Barthel Self-Care Ratings
Sherwood, S. J., Morris, J., Mor, V., & Gutkin, C. (1977). Compendium of measures for discribing and assessing long-term care population. Boston: Hebrew Rehabilitation Center for the Aged.
3. IADL & PADL
Lawton, M. P., & Brody, E. (1969). Assessment of older people: Instrumental activities of daily living. Gerontologist, (9), 179–189.
4. Rapid Disability Rating Scale
Linn, M. (1967). The rapid disability rating scale. Journal of the American Geriatrics Society, (12), 211–214.

MENTAL STATUS-COGNITIVE

1. FROMAJE
Libow, L. S. (1977). Pseudo-senility: acute and reversible organic brain syndrome. In
C. Eisdorfer & R. O. Friedel (Eds.), *Cognitive and emotional disturbance in the
elderly: Clinical issues.* Chicago: Year Book Medical Publishers.
2. Mental Status Questionnaire (MSQ)
Kahn, R. L., Goldfarb, A. I., Pollack, M., & Peck, A. (1960). Brief objective
measures for the determination of mental status in the aged. *American Journal of
Psychiatry,* (117), 326–328.

MENTAL STATUS-AFFECTIVE

1. Beck Depression Inventory
Beck, A. T., Ward, C. H., Mendelson, M., Mock, J., & Erbaugh, J. (1961). An
inventory for measuring depression. *Archives of General Psychiatry* (4), 53–63
2. Philadelphia Geriatric Center (PGC)
Morale Scale (See multidimensional)
3. Zung Self-Rating Depression Scale
Zung, W. W. K. (1965). A self-rating depression scale. *Archives of General Psychiatry,*
(12), 63–70

SOCIAL

1. Environmental Fit: Satisfaction with Nursing Home Scale
McCaffree, K. M., & Harkins, E. M. (1976). Final report for evaluation of the
outcomes of nursing home care. Seattle: Battelle Human Affairs Research Centers.
2. Locus and Range of Activities Checklist
Hulica, I., Morganti, J., & Cataldo, J. (1975). Perceived latitude of choice of institutionalized and noninstitutionalized elderly women. *Experimental Aging Research,*
(1) 27–39
3. Social Interaction. See OARS (Multidimensional)

ECONOMIC

See OARS

MULTIDIMENSIONAL

1. Philadelphia Geriatric Center: Multi-Level Assessment Instrument Manual
Write to:

M. Powell Lawton, PhD
or
Miriam S. Moss
Philadelphia Geriatric Center
5301 Old York Road
Philadelphia, Pa 19141
(215) 455-6162
2. Older Americans' Resources and Services (OARS)
Duke University. (1978). *The OARS methodology* (2nd ed.). Durham, NC: The Duke
University Center for the Study of Aging and Human Development

DEPRESSION

Beck, A. T., & Beck, R. W. (1972). Screening depressed patients in family practice:
A rapid technique. *Post-graduate Medicine, 57*, 81–85.
Brink, T., Yesavage, J., Lum, O., Heersema, P., Adey, M., & Rose, T. (1982).
Screening tests for depression. *Clinic Gerontologist, (1)*, 37–43.
Popoff, L. M. (1969). A simple method of diagnosis of depression by the family
physician. *Clinical Medicine, 76*, 24–29.
Zung, W. W. K. (1965). A self-rating depression scale. *Archives of General Psychiatry,
12*, 63–70.

STRESS

Stokes/Gordon Stress Scale
Shirlee Stokes
Pace University
Lienhard School of Nursing
Bedford Road
Pleasantville, NY 10570

APPENDIX E

Federal Council on Aging Recommendations for Mental Health Care of the Aged

A. PREVENTION

1. Effective systems for teaching the elderly to cope with the aging process should be developed. Expanded support should be given to exploring and applying effective strategies for disseminating this knowledge through the media, care providers, educational institutions, senior citizen groups, and other community organizations.

2. Programs that provide the elderly with the opportunity for new and/or continued community roles and activities should receive increased emphasis and support.

3. Increased support should be given to the development, dissemination, and expansion of effective models of preretirement and postretirement education programs, in cooperation with industry, unions, colleges, universities, and senior citizen and voluntary organizations.

4. A major program of public education should be developed to combat prejudice toward the old and to improve the image of the

aging experience in the eyes of the general public, the media, service providers, and the elderly themselves. Actions to combat age discrimination in all its aspects should be vigorously pursued.

5. To help provide appropriate services and avoid unwarranted institutionalization, a nationwide system of Comprehensive Geriatric Assessment Units should be created within existing community programs to serve as assessment, assignment, treatment, and coordinating centers on an area-wide basis.

6. Crisis intervention programs at the community level should be developed and expanded to provide services for the elderly who are at high risk of developing mental illness.

7. A comprehensive, long-term social support system should be developed in each community for elderly persons who are chronically ill, socially isolated, and/or frail which can provide, on a sustained basis, those services needed to promote and maintain maximum levels of functioning. Existing agencies and organizations should be used to the fullest extent possible, while new models must be designed and tested to ensure that present gaps in services are closed.

8. The most vulnerable groups of community dwelling elderly should be entitled to special assistance in planning for and gaining access to the services they need: the deinstitutionalized chronically mentally ill and those with severely reduced physical and emotional capacities due to extreme old age. Federal support should be given to developing and testing models for sustained community agency responsibility for regularly monitoring and ensuring needed services for these high-risk elderly.

B. SERVICES

1. In order to improve the availability and accessibility of mental health care for elderly persons, coverage for mental health services should be provided on an equal basis with coverage for physical health care services, for both acute and chronic illnesses. In existing third-party programs, current inequities in coverage for mental health care services must be redressed, making mental health care services as accessible as physical health care services, for both acute and chronic illnesses.

2. A national policy to ensure the availability of a full-range of mental health services for the elderly, ranging from ambulatory to home health, congregate living, day and/or night care, transitional care (half-way houses), foster homes, rehabilitative services, and specialized inpatient services should be developed.

3. In order to provide quality mental health services to the elderly, staff of health and mental health providing specialized services to the elderly should have specific expertise and training in geriatric mental health care. Regulations governing third-party payments to such facilities as community mental health centers or other comprehensive mental health programs, public or private mental hospitals, or university-operated or affiliated teaching hospitals should require that these institutions demonstrate adequate staff training as a condition of provider eligibility.

4. Staff development and inservice training costs should be an allowable item for Medicare and Medicaid reimbursement up to five percent of total service delivery costs.

5. In long-term care facilities, mental health services should be regularly provided to all patients having significant mental disorders, either directly by the facility or by an outside agency by written agreement.

6. A focal point should be designed at the state level to ensure that the mental health needs of the elderly are being and will be met through careful assessment, coordination, and planning of statewide health, mental health, and social services. Financial and technical assistance should be provided to states to strengthen their capacity for geriatric mental health service assessment, coordination, planning, and development.

C. RESEARCH

1. An expanded national research program on the causes, treatment, and prevention of senile dementia and on changes in intellectual functioning and/or ability in later life should be supported.

2. An expanded research effort to determine the causes, treatment, and prevention of depression in older persons including investigations of the relationships of depression to suicide, alcoholism, and other symptomatic and behavioral disorders should be initiated.

3. Actions to develop a national data base on the epidemiology and demography of mental disorders of the elderly should be undertaken.

4. Research on mental health services, delivery systems, and treatment interventions should be targeted for expanded support; such investigations should include the development of successful models and the evaluation of their effectiveness for differing populations.

5. Psychopharmacological research—investigations of the aging process as it effects differential responsiveness to drugs—should be targeted for increased Federal support.

6. Research efforts pertaining to the causation, prevention, and amelioration of the major crises of later life should receive increased emphasis and support.

7. Research investigations of the causes, effects, and ways to eliminate prejudicial attitudes toward the elderly should be expanded.

8. In order to pursue the expanded research effort described in the preceding recommendations, the capacities of existing Federal agencies to support research relevant to mental health of the elderly should be strengthened, while preserving a pluralistic, coordinated approach, especially in such areas as dementia research. While the National Institute of Mental Health should assume particular responsibilities for mental health research because of its basic mandate in this regard, the unique potentials of the National Institute on Aging and the Administration on Aging should also be enhanced.

D. TRAINING

1. A national training effort to develop faculty with expertise in geriatric mental health in the major mental health, health, and social service disciplines should be initiated.

2. A national training effort should be initiated to enhance the geriatric mental health knowledge and skill of existing service providers in the mental health, health, and social service fields.

3. Federal efforts to support the development and inclusion of geriatric mental health in the core curriculum and basic training of incoming personnel in all health, mental health, and social service disciplines should be expanded.

4. A national training effort should be supported to develop a cadre of specialists in geriatric mental health.

5. Comprehensive, Multidisciplinary Training Centers for Mental Health of the Aging should be created and supported on a regional basis. These centers should be affiliated with appropriate institutions having extensive research and service programs.

6. Content in mental health and aging should be included as a required component of continuing education in programs related to licensure, relicensure, certification, and recertification of health and mental health professionals.

E. MINORITIES

1. Federally funded research and demonstration projects should be established at selected sites throughout the country to explore meth-

ods for better serving the mental health needs of elderly minority group members and to conduct research on specific minority aging issues.

2. The development of strategies for ensuring better access to services for the elderly minority group members should be pursued by all Federal agencies.

3. Data collection systems in all Federal programs serving the elderly should include provision for reporting of age (by subcategories), sex, race, and ethnic origin.

4. The nationwide training program in mental health and illness of the elderly, recommended by the Committee, should make a substantial effort to develop specialized training for serving minorities. In addition, grants-in-aid, scholarships, and fellowship programs should be offered to stimulate minority participation in training for geriatric mental health research, service, and education.

5. Advisory groups and other bodies responsible for evaluating and initiating public programs serving minority elderly should include representation by minority specialists in the aging and mental health fields.

F. MAJOR STRATEGIES FOR IMPLEMENTATION

1. The Medicare and Medicaid legislation should be amended to extend the same coverage and benefits for mental illness that are now available for physical illness.

2. The Medicare and Medicaid legislation should be amended to place the providers of mental health services on an equal basis with the providers of general health services.

3. The quality assurance mechanisms built into Medicare and Medicaid should be strengthened to include the mental health components in staff requirements, provider qualifications, and professional review of services.

4. New benefits for all Medicare patients should be added that would be of particular value to patients with mental disorders.

5. Medicare entitlement should be extended to all recipients of Supplementary Security Income, to those who are 50 years and older and disabled.

6. The National Health Planning and Resources Development Act of 1974 should be amended to provide that Health Systems Agencies are responsible for assuring the inclusion of mental health services and resources needed by the elderly in their health systems plans and annual implementation plans.

7. Title XX of the Social Security Act should be amended to require that social support services necessary for comprehensive mental health care be a component of the state social service plan.

8. Title III of the Older Americans Act should be amended to provide that the state and area agencies on aging are responsible for the inclusion of mental health services in their state and area plans.

9. Existing legislative authorities should be used to provide expanded support to experimentation and demonstration of improved methods of delivery of mental health services.

10. Each Federal program with legislative authority to support or carry out research and/or training should devote an appropriate proportion of their efforts to problems of mental health and illness of the aging.

11. Congress should establish a National Commission on Mental Health and Illness of the Elderly.

12. The Commission should give special attention to the quality and comparability of statistical data on the aged (e.g., their health, mental health, and social status and needs, and types and costs of health and mental health services utilized) that are now collected by each of the Federal programs concerned with the general health and mental health needs of the aging population.

APPENDIX F

Resources and Tools for Assessing the Elderly

MONITORING WANDERING BEHAVIORS

Fennelly, Andrew L.
Secure Care Systems, Inc.
P.O. Box 1180
Portland, ME 04104

RELAXATION

Holistic Nursing Practice (Quarterly Journal)
Aspen Publishers
7201 McKinney Circle
Frederick, MD 21701

Autogenic Health Center
6401 Broadway Terrace
Oakland, CA 94618

National Center for the Exploration of Human Potential
6731 Bamhurst St.
San Diego, CA 92117

Stamford Center for the Healing Arts
First Congregational Church
Walton Place
Stamford, CT 06901

Institute for Psychoenergetics
126 Harvard St.
Brookline, MA 02146

RESOURCES

Producer of documentary films on aging and other subjects.
Tom Hotchkiss
Tri-Media Communications
Boise, ID.

Provides sex information to older persons as well as others.
SEICUS
Sex Information and Education Council of the United States
84 Fifth Ave, Suite 407
New York, N.Y. 10011

Gerontologic Practitioners in nursing homes.
Audry Smith-Gerontologic Nurse Practitioner
GNP
Boise Samaritan Village
Boise, ID

Resource for Remotivation
Kits available from the American Psychiatric Association, Washington, D.C. and a film, *Remotivation. A New Technique for the Psychiatric Aide*, is available from:
Film Center
Services Department
Smith Kline and French Laboratories
1500 Spring Garden St.
Philadelphia, PA 19101

Dorothy Smith originated the remotivation technique while working as a volunteer in a mental hospital. Later, in 1956, she trained a large group at Pennsylvania State Hospital in the use of remotivation techniques (Long, 1962).

Environmental adaptation
Chalet Nursing Home, Yakima WN

Information about developing "Travel day" in a nursing home
Sister Lucia Gamroth
Benedictine Nursing Center
Mt. Angel, Oregon

Other facilities that have travel days:
Desert Life Health Center in Tucson, AZ
Bethany Home, Ripon, CA
La Mesa Convalescent Center, La Mesa, CA
Manzana del Sol in Albuquerque, NM
WestSide Medical Center, VA, Chicago, IL

Resources and educational materials for elders and their caregivers

American Association of Retired Persons
AARP Health Advocacy Services
1909 K St., NW
Washington, DC 70049

Long Distance Family Caregiving
Nancy Wexler
Management of Problems of Middle Aged Adults and Their Parents
Tarzana, CA

Index